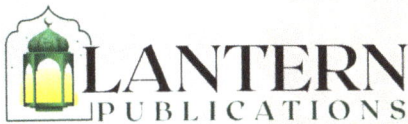

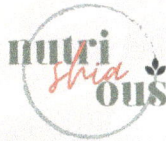

Lantern Publications
info@lanternpublications.com
www.lanternpublications.com
Instagram: @lanternpublications

Nutrishiaous
nutrishiaous.company.site
nutrishiaous@gmail.com
Instagram: @nutrishiaous

Ordering Information:
Quantity sales. Special discounts are available on quantity purchases by corporations, associations, and others. If you would like more details, please contact the distributor at the address below.

Shia Books
Australia-www.shiabooks.com.au
Canada-www.shiabookscanada.com
info@shiabooks.com.au

ISBN- 978-1-922583-69-7

First Edition

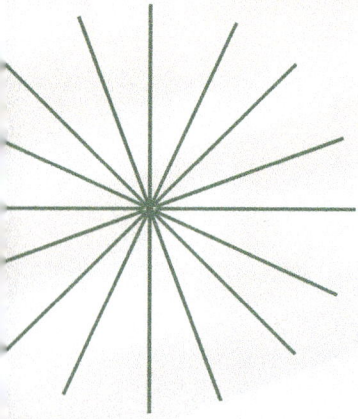

Table of Contents

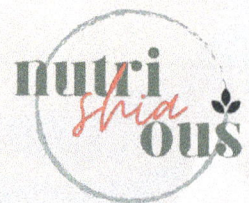

nutri shia ous

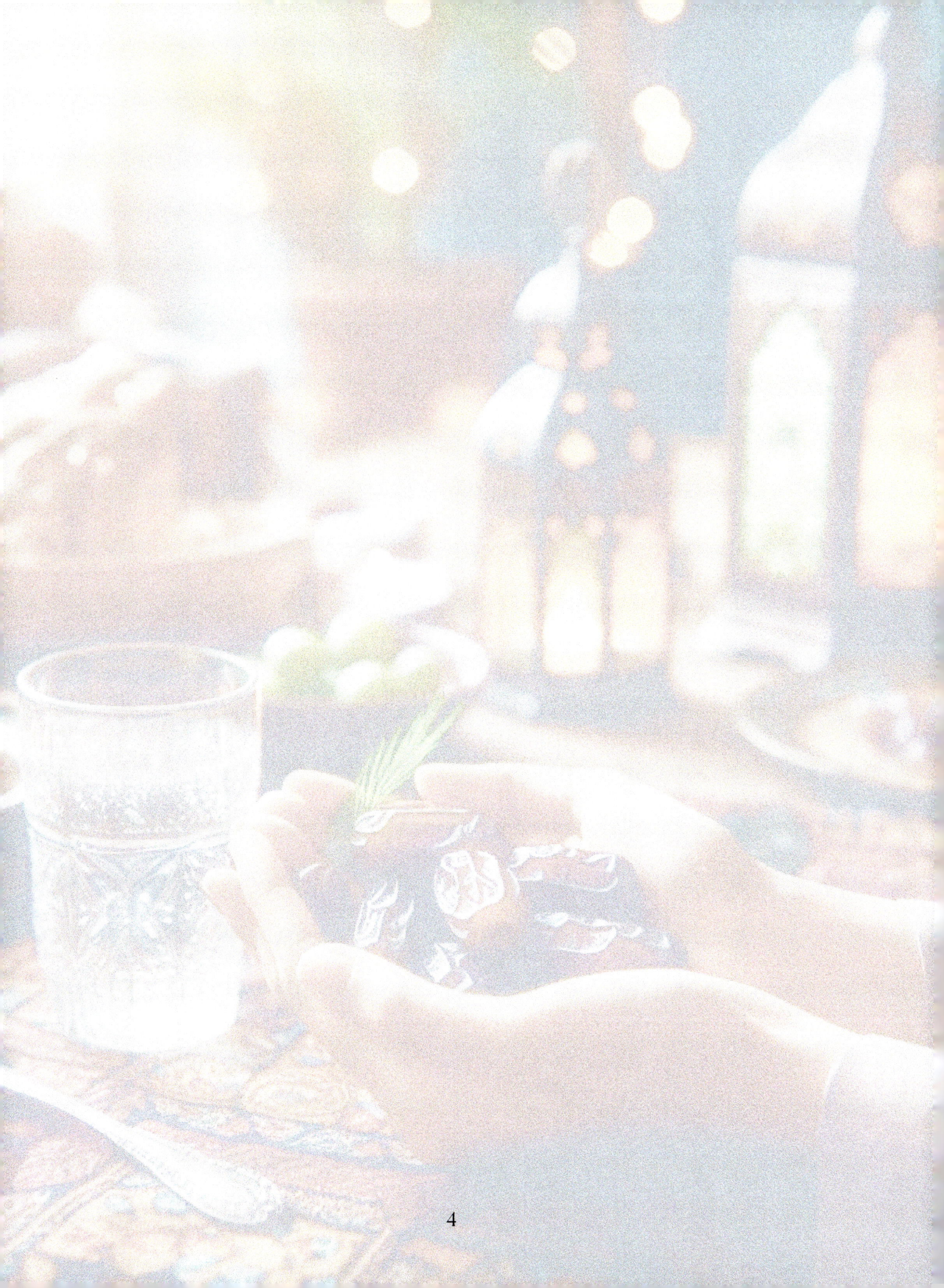

Glossary *Terms*

General Arabic Terms used in this booklet:

- <u>Shahr Ramaḍān</u> - The 7th month of the Islamic lunar calendar, in which Muslims are obligated to fast.
- <u>Ahlulbayt</u> - The family of Prophet Muḥammad (sawa).
- <u>A`immah</u> - Plural of Imam (leader), referring to the Imams of the Ahlulbayt (as).
- <u>Mustaḥab</u> - Recommended
- <u>Ma'ṣūmīn</u> - The Infallibles (i.e the Ahlulbayt)
- <u>Amīr al-Mu`minīn</u> - The Commander of the Believers (i.e Imam Ali (as))
- (<u>swt</u>) - Glory be to Him
- (<u>sawa</u>) - Peace be upon him and his family
- (<u>as</u>) - Peace be upon him/her/them

The Islamic literature this booklet will quote from:

- <u>Al-Kāfī</u> by Shaykh Muḥammad ibn Ya'qūb al-Kulaynī
- <u>Al-Maḥāsin</u> by Shaykh Abū Ja'far Aḥmad ibn Muḥammad al-Barqī
- <u>Wasā`il al-Shia</u> by Shaykh Ḥur al-'Āmilī
- <u>Kanz al-'Ummāl</u> by Ali ibn 'Abd-al-Malik ("Al-Muttaqī") al-Hindī
- <u>Mafātīḥ al-Jinān</u> by Shaykh 'Abbās al-Qummī

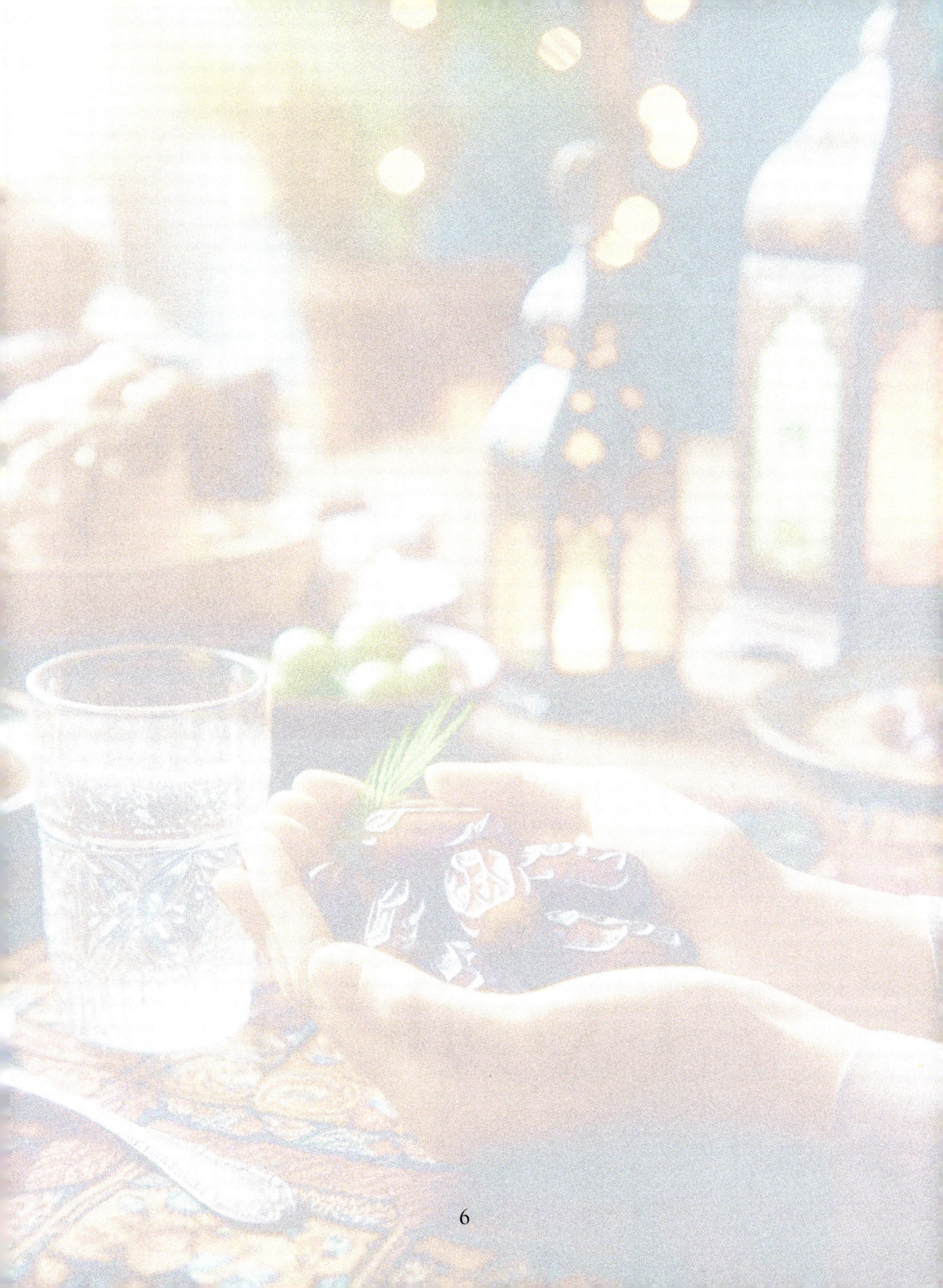

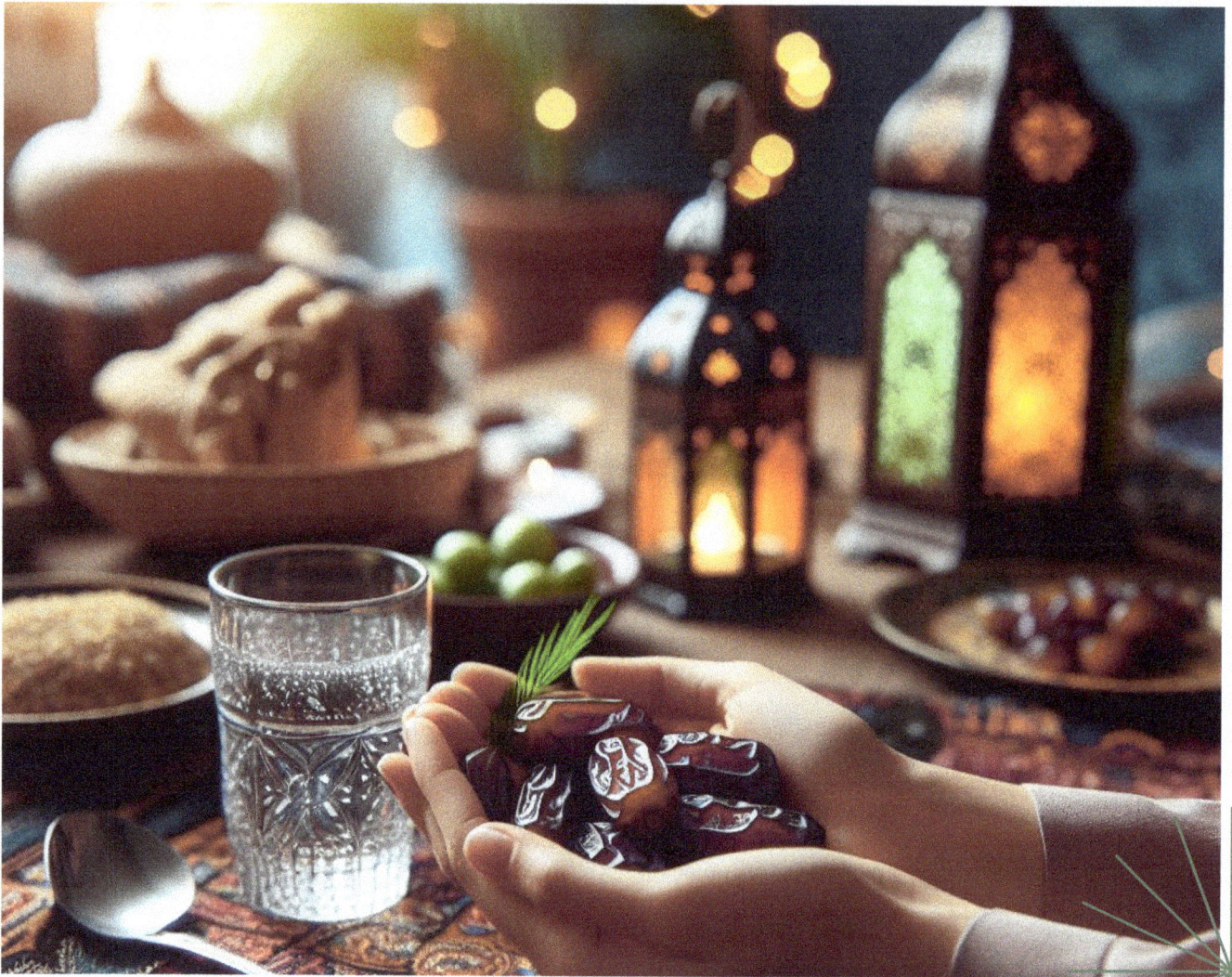

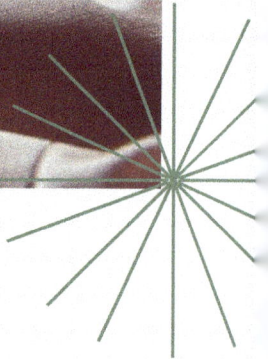

benefits of
Fasting

Spiritual BENEFITS OF FASTING

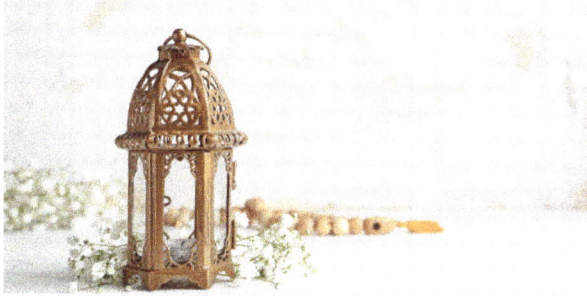

Fasting is one of the most encouraged acts of worship in Islām. During the month of Ramaḍān, Muslims must fast for 30 days, abstaining from food and drink from dawn until dark. This practice serves multiple purposes: gratitude, self-restraint, empathy, and strengthening the spiritual connection with the Almighty (swt).

Among the lowest of the benefits of fasting is its health benefits. This act is one of the main pillars of our religion. Imām al-Bāqir (as) said, "Islām is founded on five pillars. It is founded on Ṣalāt (prayer), Zakāt (charity), al-Ḥajj (pilgrimage to Mecca), fasting and our Wilāyah (love and belief in the divine authority of the Ahlulbayt). [1]"

The Prophet (sawa) said, "Fasting is incumbent upon you, for surely it severs the roots [of desires] and removes wildness. [2]" The 6th Imam also emphasized the significance of fasting, stating that "The Zakāt (cleansing of the body) is fasting. [3]" Furthermore, he stated, "The sleep of a fast observer is regarded as worship; his silence is considered praise, his deeds are accepted and his supplications are granted. [4]"

In a speech delivered on the last Friday before the month of Ramaḍān, the Holy Prophet (sawa) reminded, "With your thirst and hunger remind yourself about the thirst and hunger of the Day of Judgement; pay charity to poor people, pay respect to elders; be kind towards youngsters, and observe the bonds of relationship with your kith and kins. [5]" Furthermore, Amīr al-Mu`minīn (as) said, "Fasting of the heart is better than the fasting of the tongue, and fasting of the tongue is better than the fasting of the stomach."

1] al-Kāfī, Vol. 4, Chp. 1, Ḥadīth 1
2] Kanz al-'Ummāl, no. 23610
3] al-Kāfī, Vol. 4, Ḥadith 2
4] Wasā`il al-Shia, Vol. 7, Pg. 294
5] Wasā`il al-Shia, Vol. 7, Pg. 227

BENEFITS TO METABOLISM AND GENERAL HEALTH

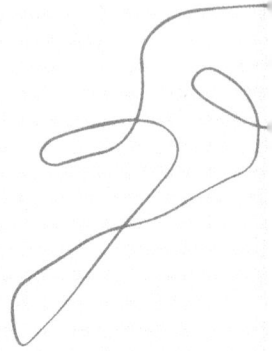

From a medical and scientific perspective, fasting can promote weight loss by burning fat more effectively and boosting metabolism [1]. Fasting has also been shown to reduce inflammation. A study in 2019 found that it helps reduce body inflammation and enhance the body's defences against oxidative and metabolic stress [2]

A review in the journal Nutrients showed that fasting can boost the immune system. It found that intermittent fasting improves immune parameters and reduces intestinal inflammation, helping the body to fight off infections better and maintain overall health [3]. Another study revealed that fasting reduced body weight, improved glucose metabolism, lowered blood pressure and enhanced lipid profiles, which are key factors in improving cardiovascular health [4].

Furthermore, fasting has many mental health benefits, associated with improved mental well-being and a reduction in symptoms of depression [5]. These psychological benefits may arise from the profound spiritual experiences during this sacred month.

1] Migala, J. (2021, March 5). The benefits of fasting for metabolic health. Levels.com; Levels. https://www.levels.com/blog/the-benefits-of-fasting-for-metabolic-health

2] de Cabo, R., & Mattson, M. P. (2019). Effects of Intermittent Fasting on Health, Aging, and Disease. New England Journal of Medicine, 381(26), 2541–2551. https://doi.org/10.1056/nejmra1905136

3] Haasis, E., Bettenburg, A., & Lorentz, A. (2024). Effect of Intermittent Fasting on Immune Parameters and Intestinal Inflammation. Nutrients, 16(22), 3956. https://doi.org/10.3390/nu16223956

4] Qiu, Z., Yun, E., Li, Y., Xiao, Y., Fu, Y., Du, J., & Kan, J. (2024). Beneficial effects of time-restricted fasting on cardiovascular disease risk factors: a meta-analysis. BMC Cardiovascular Disorders, 24(1). https://doi.org/10.1186/s12872-024-03863-6

5] Ajmera, R., & Jones, J. (2023, September 22). 8 Health Benefits of Fasting, Backed by Science. Healthline; Healthline Media. https://www.healthline.com/nutrition/fasting-benefits

PORTION CONTROL

Portion control during Shahr Ramaḍān is essential for maintaining a balanced diet and overall well-being. By managing portion sizes, individuals can avoid overeating and ensure they consume a variety of nutrients necessary for sustained energy throughout the day. This practice supports physical health and enhances the spiritual experience of fasting.

1 **Plan your meals from before**: This is where meal planning comes into play! It helps avoid indecisiveness, and impulsive eating and allows you to have balanced meals.

2 **Use a smaller plate**: This tricks your brain into thinking you are eating more than you are.

3 **Eat slowly**: It is very easy to lose control and eat quickly, as soon as you break your fast. Consciously remind yourself to eat slower, so your body can recognize its fullness cues.

4 **Start with a light meal soup or salad**: This can help fill you up and prevent you from overeating.

5 **Avoid extreme sugary items and fried foods:** It is very easy to reach for that spring roll or samosa in your hunger, but this can lead to weight gain, and heaviness after eating. Try using healthier cooking methods like baking or air frying to limit oil use or opt for healthier options!

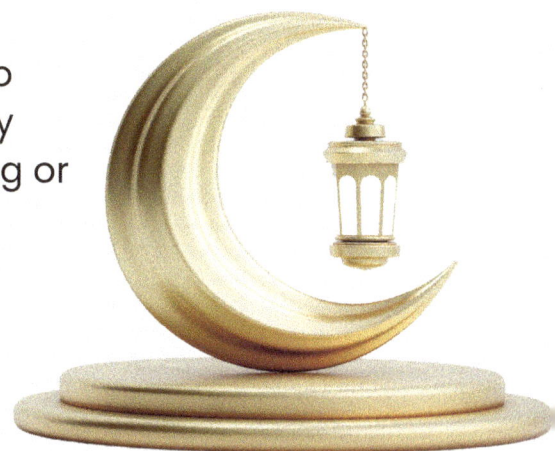

EXERCISE + NUTRITION

It is crucial to balance our nutrition with exercise, especially in this month.

1 **Time your workouts** right before Suhūr or after Iftār to ensure you have energy and are hydrated. Avoid intense exercise during the day to prevent fatigue or dehydration.

2 Save your high-intensity workouts for times when you can replenish with a meal. During the fasting hours, focus on **moderate exercise** like yoga, walking, or light strength training.

3 **Don't push yourself!** Pay attention to how you feel to avoid feeling exhausted or dizzy.

4 **Be consistent!** A consistent schedule can have many benefits like managing stress and improving your wellbeing.

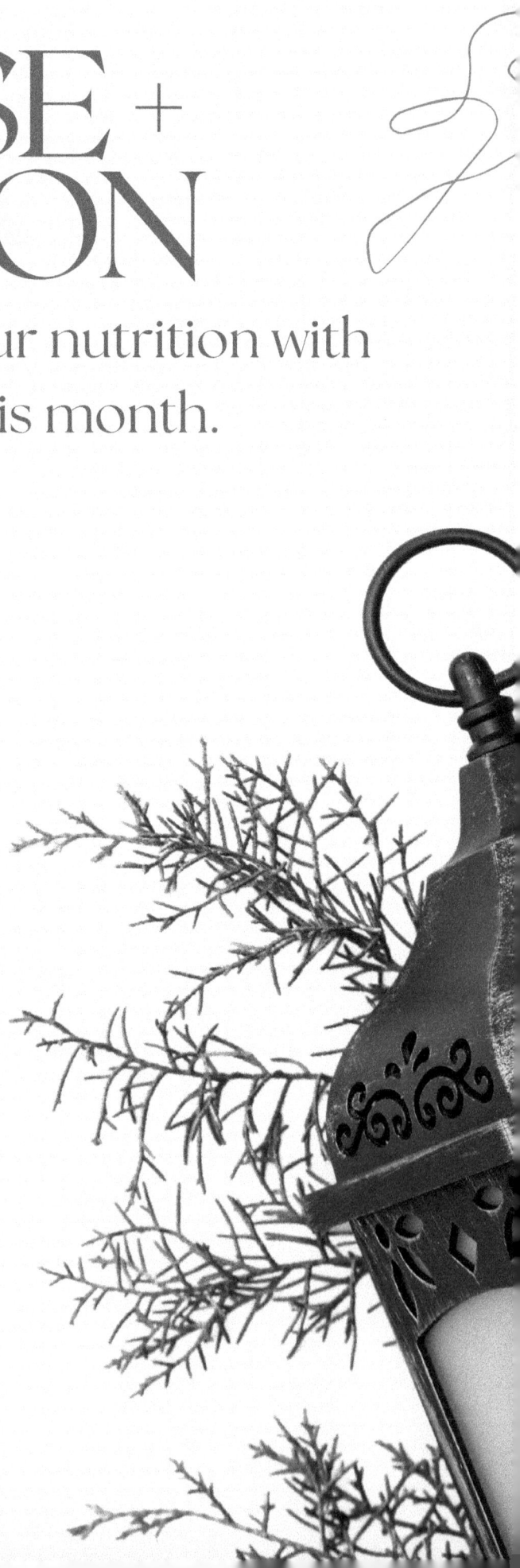

11

TIPS FOR SPECIAL DIETARY NEEDS

Diabetes:
Choose complex carbohydrates (whole grains and legumes) to allow a slow release of energy throughout the day. It is crucial to monitor your blood sugar levels throughout the day and consult your family doctor to ensure you are healthy.

Gastrointestinal Issues:
Fatty or spicy foods may trigger your symptoms or make them worse. Avoid those and stick to smaller, more frequent meals (during non-fasting periods).

High cholesterol:
Incorporate healthy fats (olive oil, avocado, nuts etc.) into your meals and avoid trans fats or saturated fats (found in red meat or full-fat dairy products). Also consume fibre-rich foods (beans, oats, lentils etc.).

Hypertension:
Limit the consumption of salty foods. Make sure to use herbs and spices to flavour your food.

Heart Disease:
Your diet should consist of healthy fats which are found in fish, nuts, seeds and olive oil. Limit your salt intake and avoid a diet high in saturated or trans fats.

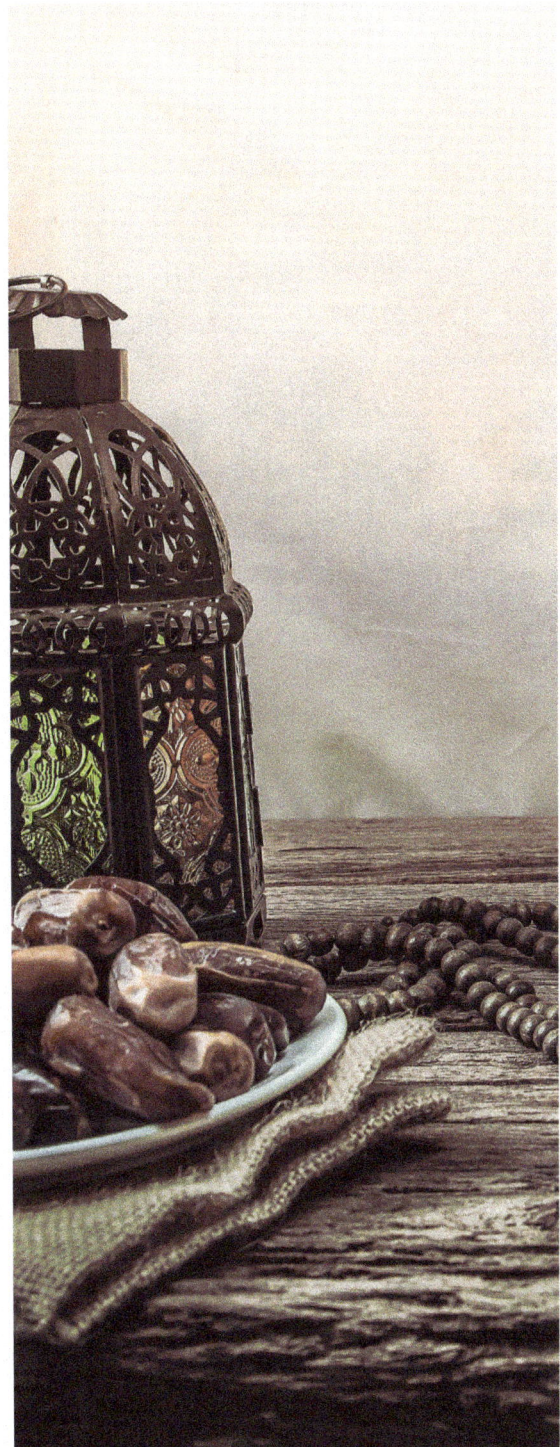

BENEFITS OF USING *supplements* DURING THIS MONTH

Supplements can be beneficial during the fasting month however, it is best to consult with a doctor on what is best for you. Here are some things to consider:

PROBIOTICS

Found in foods like yogurt and in capsule form, probiotics should be taken at Suḥūr or Iftār to maintain good gut health.

ELECTROLYTES

Sodium, potassium, and magnesium maintain fluid balance, muscle function, and cellular function. They also aid in keeping you hydrated. Have these at Suḥūr time, and again at Iftār if you notice you have extreme thirst or your body does not retain water well.

MULTI-VITAMINS

These should be taken at Suḥūr time, to allow for nutrient absorption. Take a blood test before Shahr Ramaḍān to see if you are deficient in any vitamins or minerals. Based on that, take any additional supplements like Vitamin D, C or Iron etc.

hydration BEFORE & AFTER FASTING TIMES

promotes digestive health

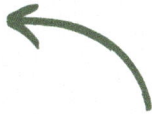

prevents dehydration

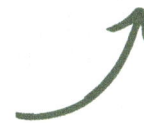

regulates body temperature

ensures energy levels remain

supports kidney function

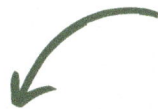

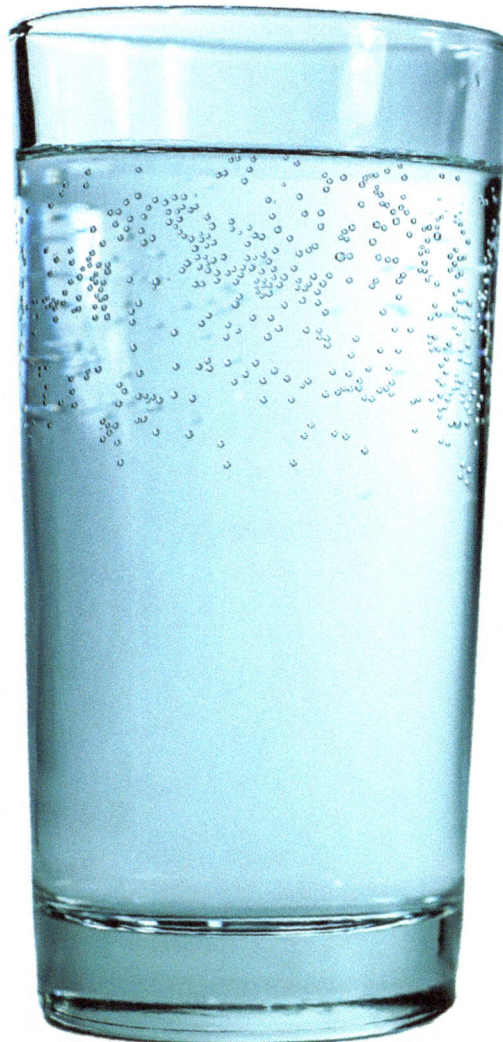

essential for cognitive function

OTHER OPTIONS

Water should be the first choice, but other options include **smoothies**, **coconut water** and/or **herbal teas**

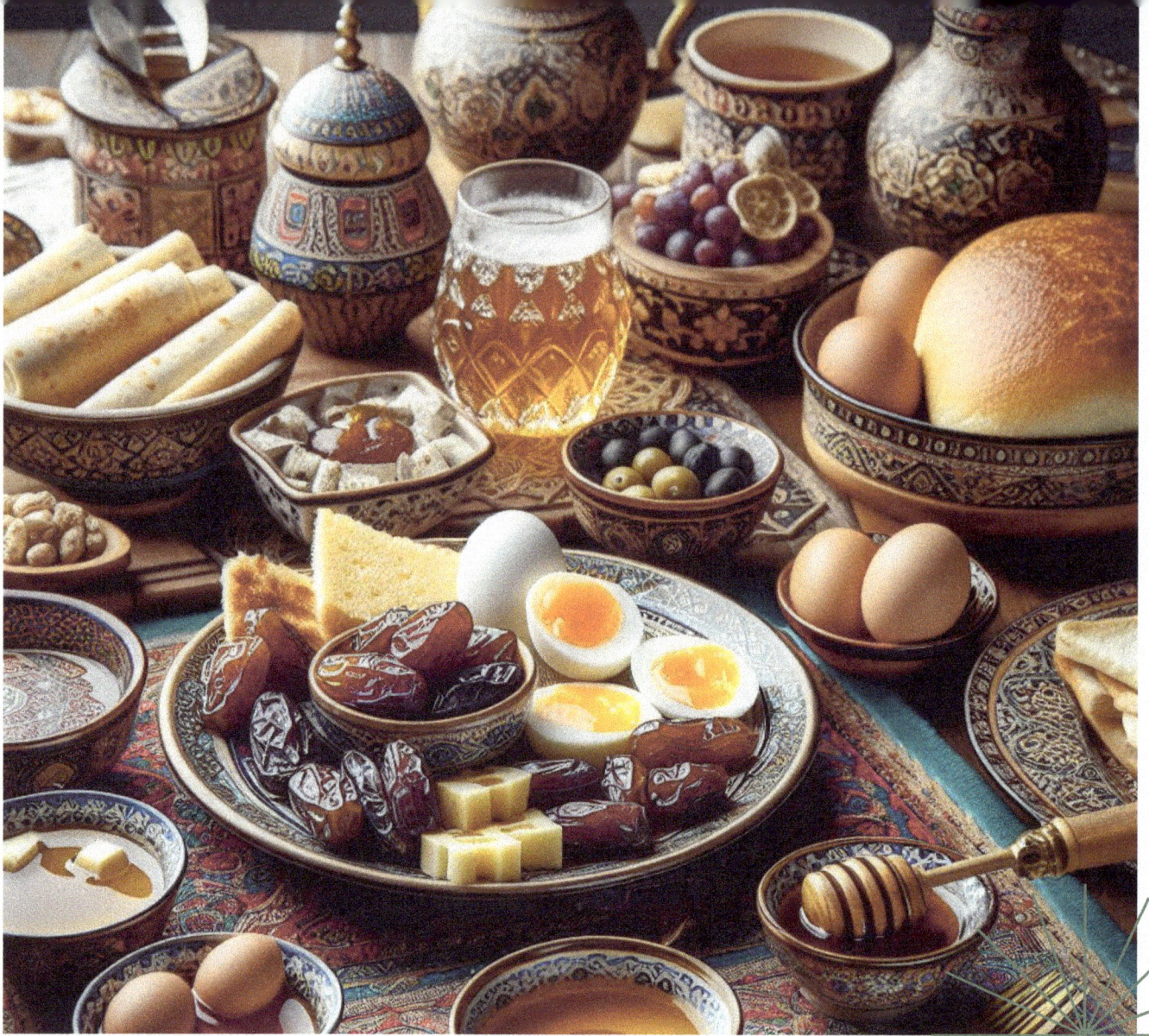

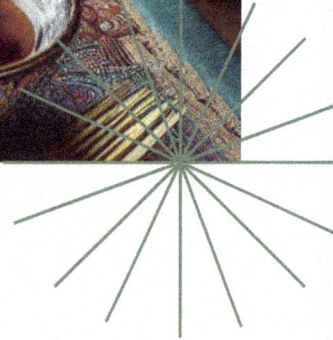

pre-dawn meal

Suḥūr

SUHŪR: A CRUCIAL NECCESSITY

Suhūr, the pre-dawn meal before fasting (especially during the month of Ramaḍān), has been highly encouraged by the Maʿṣūmīn (as).

Imam al-Ṣādiq (as) said, "Breakfast before dawn (Suhūr) is a blessing." [1]

It holds great significance in maintaining energy levels and one's overall well-being during Shahr Ramaḍān. The Ahlulbayt (as) have urged having a bite to eat, even if it consists of one date or a sip of water. They have also acknowledged that some do not prefer eating before dawn, however, it is better not to ignore it in the month of Ramaḍān [2].

Certain foods have been recommended more than others, including eating something sweet and drinking water. In one narration, the Imam stated that consuming these has many benefits including cleansing the stomach and liver, preventing bad breath and easing varicose veins [3].

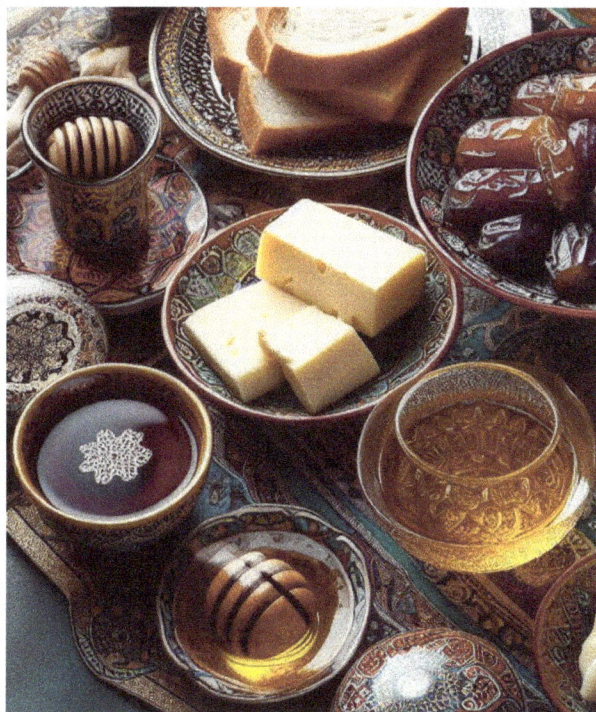

Some narrations state that the best meal is with fine flour and dates [4].

The 6th Imam emphasized its value and the Holy Prophet (sawa) advised against ignoring Suhūr. Beyond physical nourishment, Suhūr carries much spiritual significance. It has many nutritional benefits including providing energy throughout the day, hydrating the body and ensuring the body receives its required nutrients.

1] al-Kāfī, Vol. 4, Chp. 14, Ḥadīth 3
2] al-Kāfī, Vol. 4, Chp. 14, Ḥadīth 1
3] al-Kāfī, Vol. 4, Chp. 66, Ḥadīth 4
4] Mafātīḥ al-Jinān

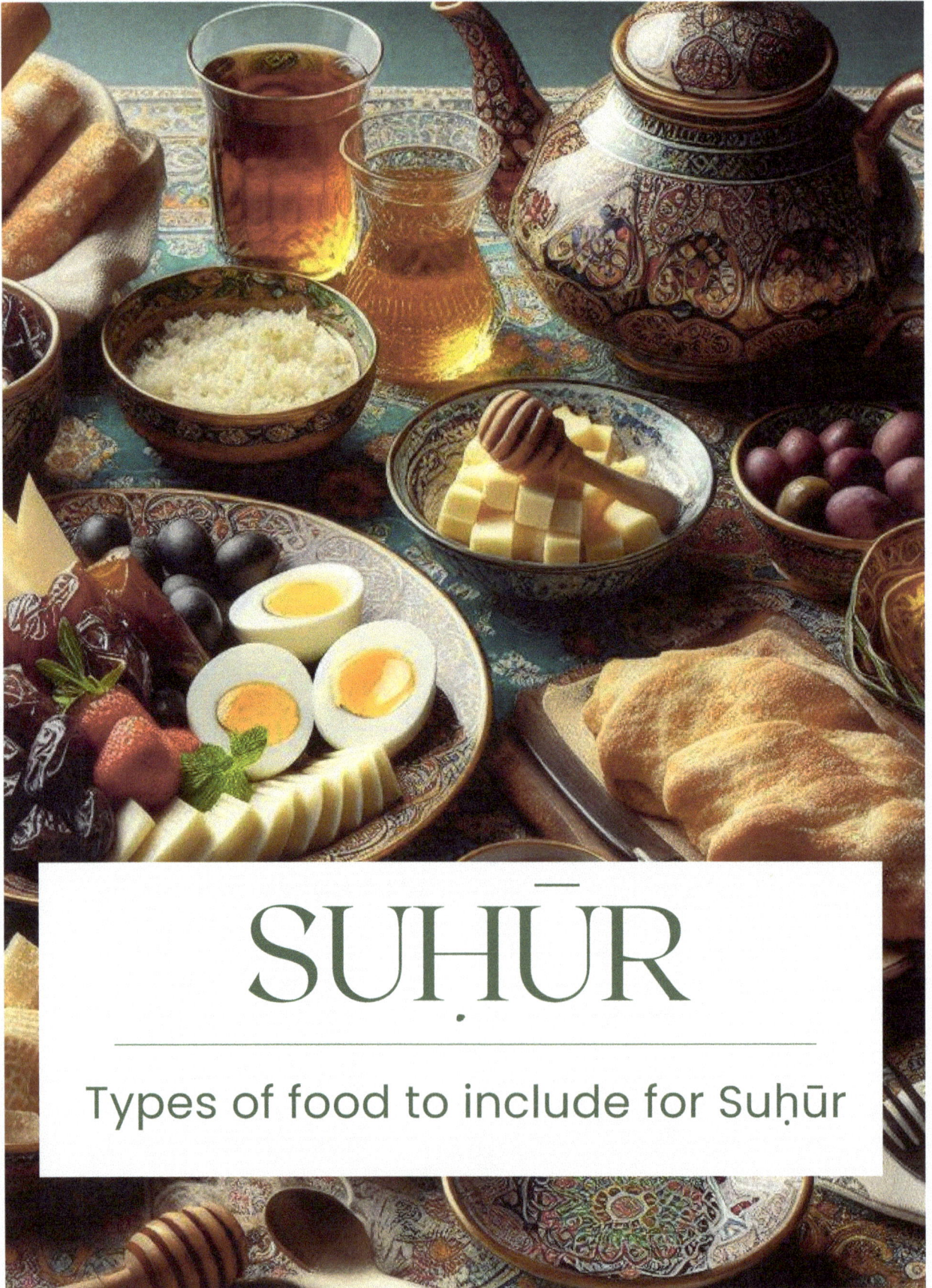

SUḤŪR

Types of food to include for Suḥūr

TYPES OF FOODS TO INCLUDE IN YOUR SUHŪR

soluble fibre

These help regulate blood sugar levels and promote digestive health.

Foods like: oats, beans, lentils, and fruits

protein

Protein supports muscle maintenance and helps control hunger.

Foods like: Eggs, yogurt, cheese or lean meats

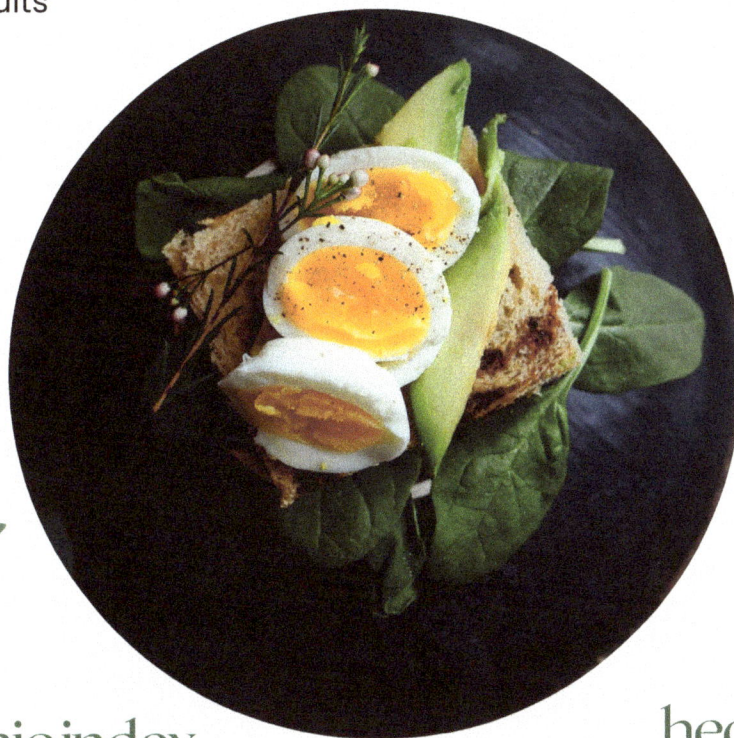

low glycemic index (GI) foods

These foods provide energy throughout the day and prevent hunger during fasting.

Foods like: Whole grains (oats, brown rice, quinoa) and whole wheat bread

healthy fats

These fats contribute to satiety and slow down digestion, keeping you full for longer.

Foods like: Healthy fats such as avocados, nuts, seeds, and olive oil.

DATES

The A`immah (as) have spoken highly of dates, stating they remove illnesses, take away fatigue, dissolve phlegm and satisfy one's hunger [1].

They are rich in fibre, high in antioxidants, provide crucial vitamins, and most importantly, are an excellent energy source.

_____

1] al-Kāfi, Vol. 6, Chp 97
2] Uddin, M. S., & Nuri, Z. N. (2021). Nutritional values and pharmacological importance of date fruit (Phoenix dactylifera Linn): A review. Journal of Current Research in Food Science, 2(1), 27-30.

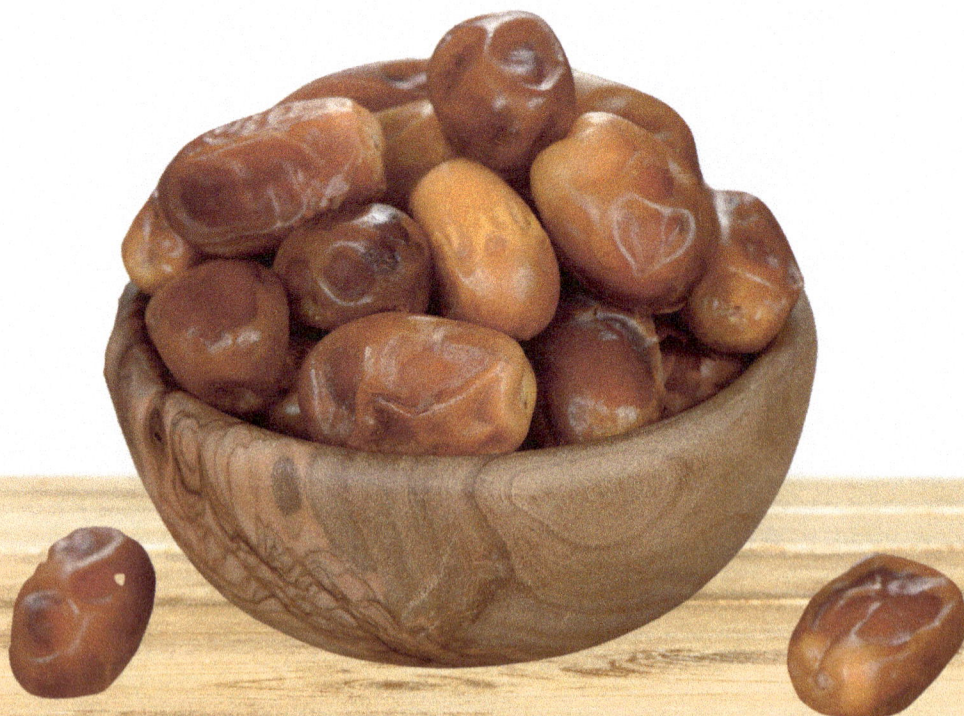

FIGS

Figs have been mentioned in the Qur`ān and spoken about by the Ahlulbayt (as). The fruit is associated with removing bad breath [1], (perfect for before fasting a long day). Furthermore, it strengthens the bones and teeth, promotes hair growth and dispels illness.

From a nutritional aspect, figs contain large amounts of fibre which supports digestive health and feeling full all day. They also have crucial vitamins and antioxidants for wellbeing [2].

1] [al-Kāfī, Vol. 6, Bk. 5, Chp 104, Ḥadith 1
2] Sandhu, A. K., Islam, M., Edirisinghe, I., & Burton-Freeman, B. (2023). Phytochemical Composition and Health Benefits of Figs (Fresh and Dried): A Review of Literature from 2000 to 2022. Nutrients, 15(11), 2623. https://doi.org/10.3390/nu15112623

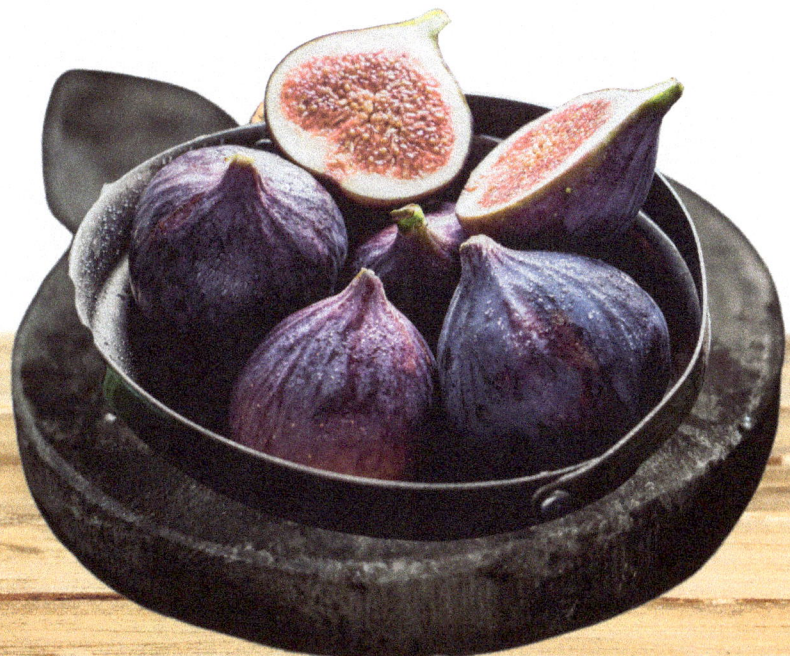

EGGS

Eggs are another filling choice for Suḥūr and are a highly Mustaḥab food by the Ahlulbayt (as). They have explained that the yolk is lighter, while the egg whites are heavier, thus more filling [1].

From a nutritional aspect, eggs are a complete protein, containing all the amino acids essential for muscle repair and overall health [2]. They are packed with Vitamins like A, B12, B2, D and E, various minerals and can reduce the risk of heart disease [3]. Lastly, the protein and fat content in eggs can provide satiety (feeling full) for longer.

1] al-Kāfī, Vol. 6, Bk. 5, Chp 75, Ḥadith 5]
2] Warner, L. (2024, December 5). Eggs, protein, and cholesterol: How to make eggs part of a heart-healthy diet - Harvard Health. Harvard Health. https://www.health.harvard.edu/nutrition/eggs-protein-and-cholesterol-how-to-make-eggs-part-of-a-heart-healthy-diet
3] Mortensen, M. B., & Nordestgaard, B. G. (2020). Elevated LDL cholesterol and increased risk of myocardial infarction and atherosclerotic cardiovascular disease in individuals aged 70–100 years: a contemporary primary prevention cohort. The Lancet, 396(10263), 1644–1652. https://doi.org/10.1016/s0140-6736(20)32233-9

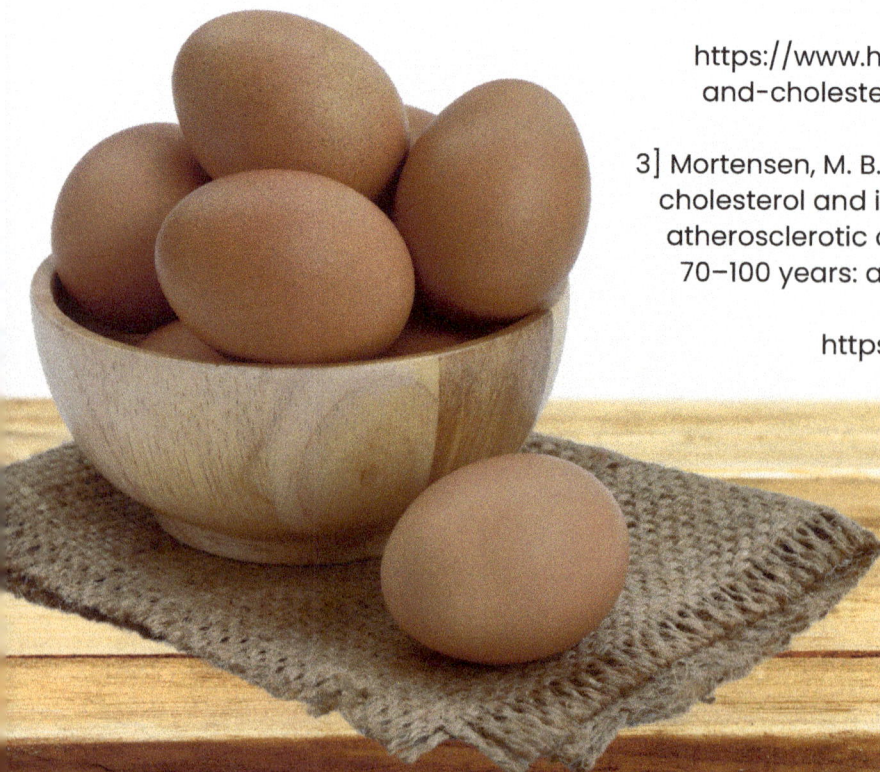

YOGURT

The Holy Prophet (sawa) and his blessed family (as) have spoken of the excellence of milk, as well as milk products from cows. Its benefits include growing flesh, strengthening the bones and acting as a form of medicine [1].

Yogurt is high in calcium, which in turn supports bone and dental health. It is high in protein, contains 8 vitamins and minerals and is extremely beneficial for gut help [2]. Prebiotics found in yogurt have also been shown to boost immune function, which can prevent individuals from getting sick [3].

1] al-Kāfī, Vol. 6, Bk. 5, Chp 84, Ḥadith 7
2] Kok, C. R., & Hutkins, R. (2018). Yogurt and other fermented foods as sources of health-promoting bacteria. Nutrition Reviews, 76(Supplement_1), 4–15. https://doi.org/10.1093/nutrit/nuy056
3] Mofid, V., Izadi, A., Mojtahedi, S. Y., & Khedmat, L. (2019). Therapeutic and Nutritional Effects of Synbiotic Yogurts in Children and Adults: a Clinical Review. Probiotics and Antimicrobial Proteins. https://doi.org/10.1007/s12602-019-09594-x

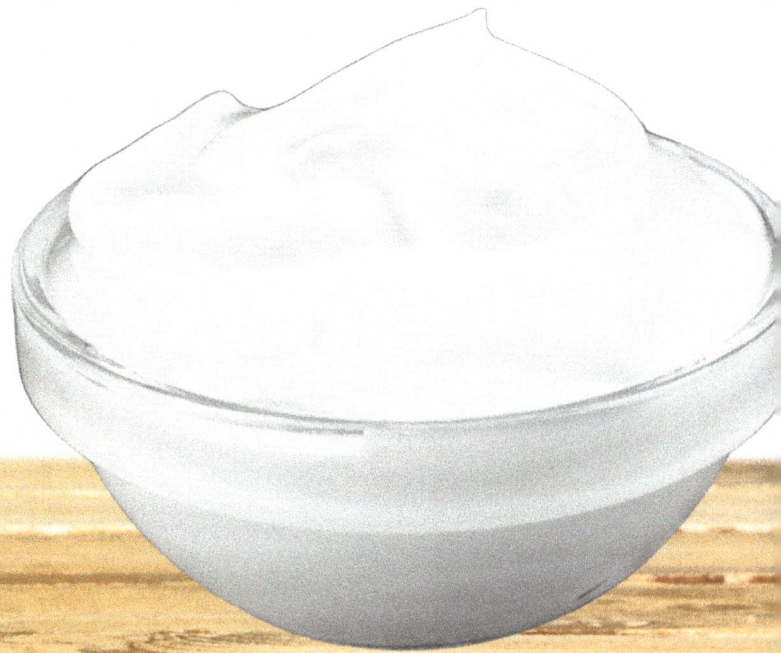

OTHER MUSTAHAB FOODS

perfect for suhūr

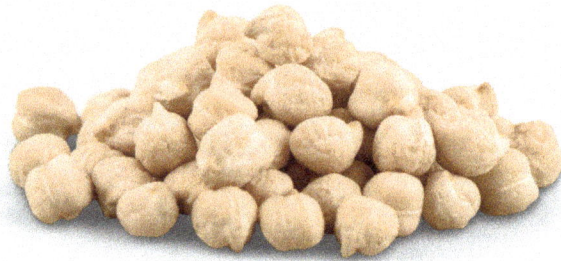

chickpeas

Chickpeas provide complex carbohydrates and protein to ensure sustained energy throughout the day.

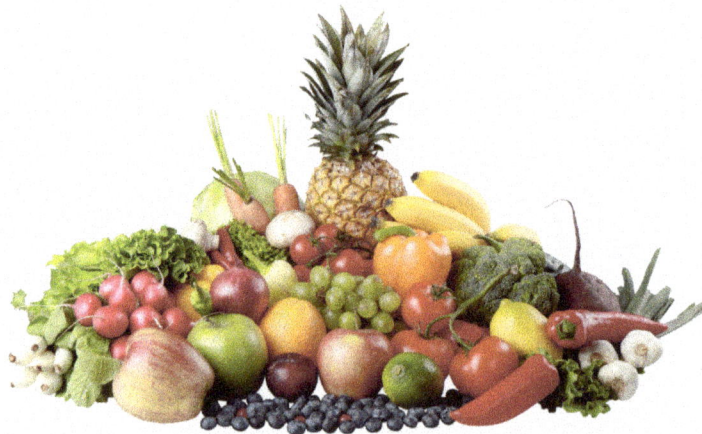

fruits

Fruits like apples, berries and oranges are packed with fibre to keep you hydrated for a long day of fasting.

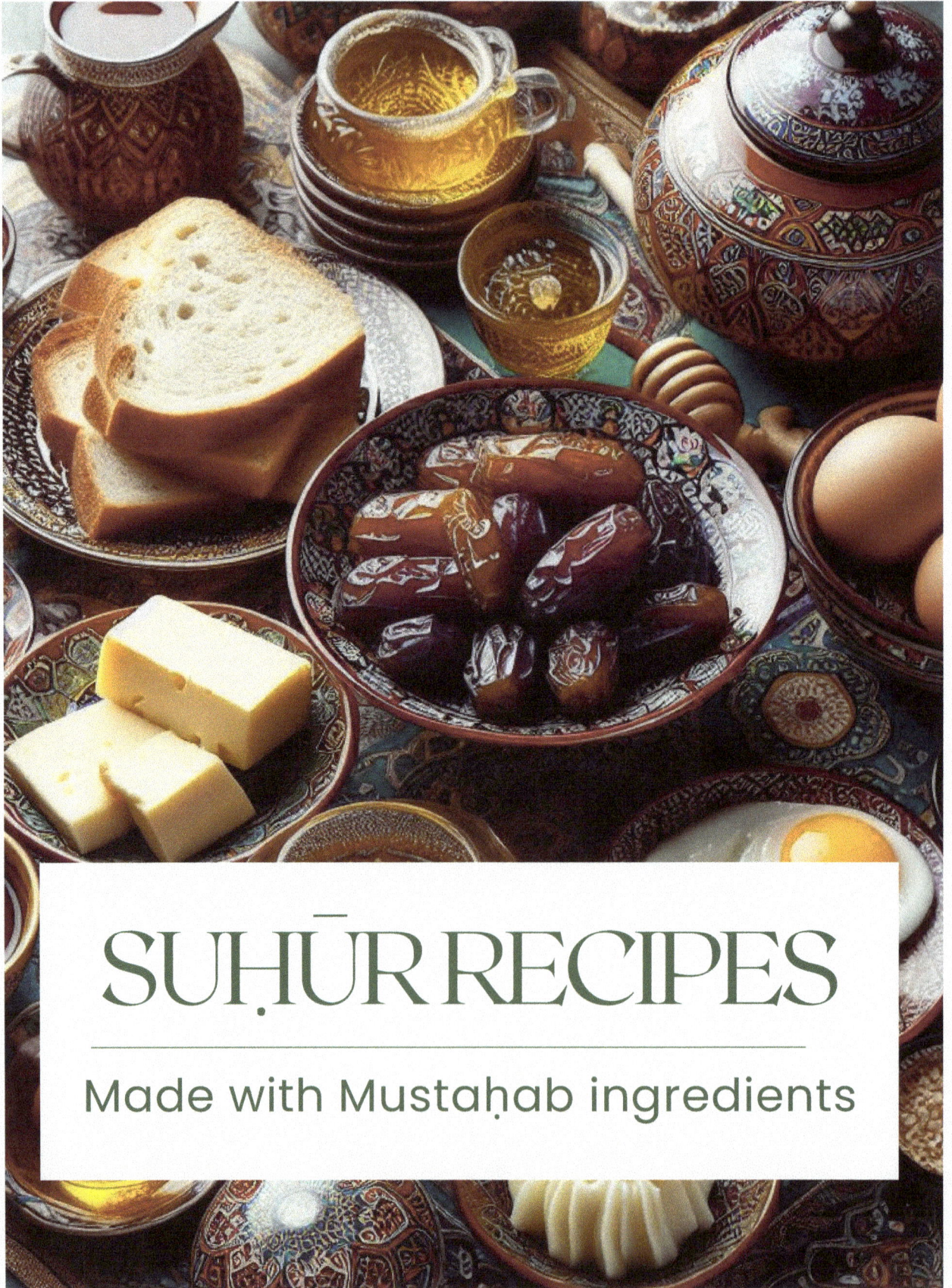

SUḤŪR RECIPES

Made with Mustaḥab ingredients

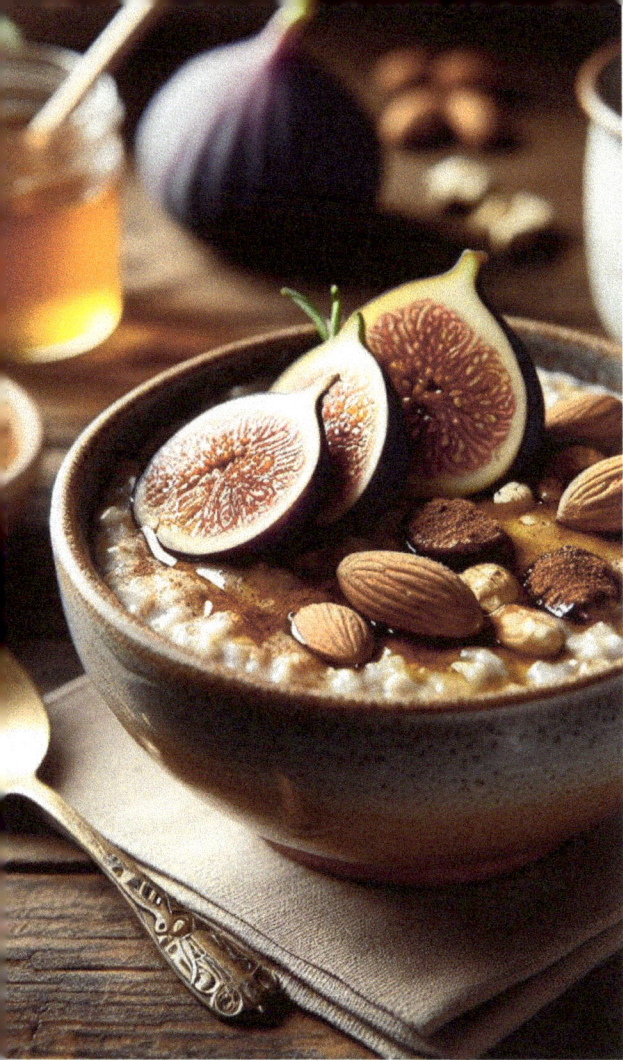

FIG AND ALMOND OVERNIGHT OATS

This is a quick meal you can make before hand and save in the fridge for a couple of days!

PREP TIME 2 MINS

COOK TIME 3 MINS

SERVINGS 1 JAR

Instructions

1. In a Mason jar or resealable container, combine the oats, milk, chopped dried figs, and almond butter.
2. Add a drizzle of honey or maple syrup if you prefer a sweeter taste.
3. Stir well to mix all the ingredients.
4. Cover the jar and refrigerate it overnight. In the morning, give it a good stir and enjoy!

Ingredients

- ½ cup old-fashioned rolled oats
- ½ cup milk (or an alternative)
- 2 dried figs, chopped
- 1 tbsp chopped almonds
- 1 tsp honey or maple syrup (for added sweetness)
- A pinch of ground cinnamon (optional)

Notes:
- Mustaḥab foods included: Figs, Milk, Almonds and Honey.
- This recipe can be adjusted and recreated with any other fruits (berries, mango, banana etc.)

26

MAPLE SWEET POTATO PANCAKES

These wholesome pancakes are fluffy, naturally sweetened and flavourful!

PREP TIME
10 MINS

COOK TIME
10 MINS

SERVINGS
1 PLATE

Instructions

1. Bake a medium sweet potato until soft (20 mins).
2. At the same time, in a small bowl, combine 2 tablespoons of maple syrup with diced apple. Set aside. Scoop out the flesh of the baked sweet potato into a small bowl. Add 2 large eggs and a pinch of salt to the sweet potato. Mash and stir until well combined.
3. Heat a large nonstick skillet over medium-high heat. Add the batter in 1/4 cup portions, leaving space between each pancake. Cook until browned on the bottom, about 3 minutes. Gently flip with a flat spatula and cook until the second side is browned, about 3 minutes more. Transfer to a plate and repeat with the remaining batter.
4. Top sweet potato pancakes with the apple-maple mixture.

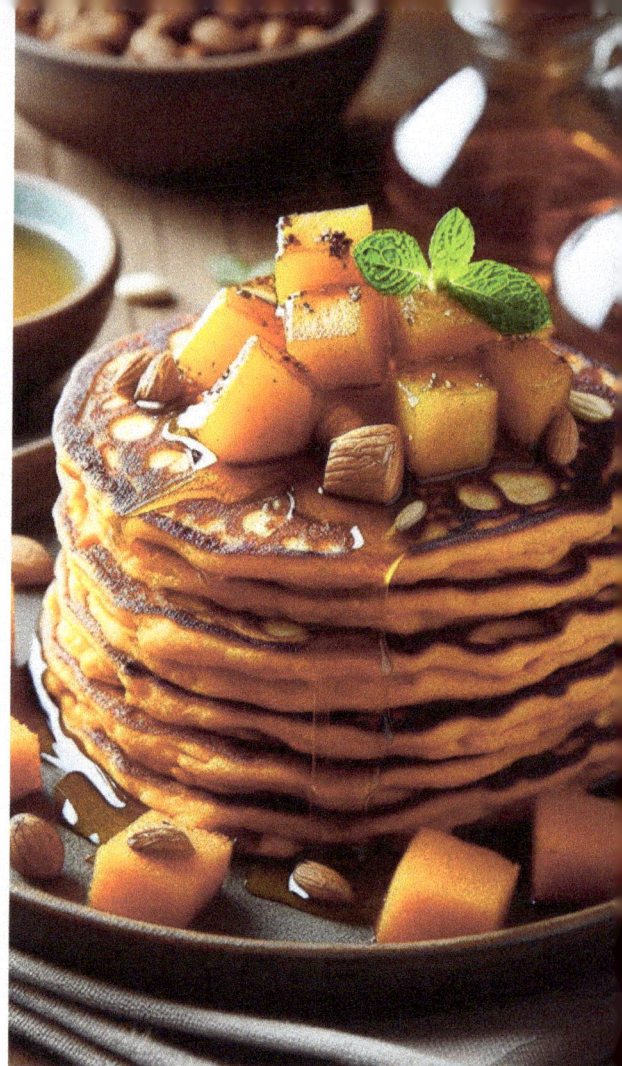

Ingredients

- 1 small apple, diced
- 2 tbsp maple syrup
- 1 baked and cooled medium sweet potato (scooped out)
- 2 large eggs
- A pinch of salt
- Coconut oil or other neutral oil for cooking

Notes:
- Mustaḥab foods included: apple and eggs

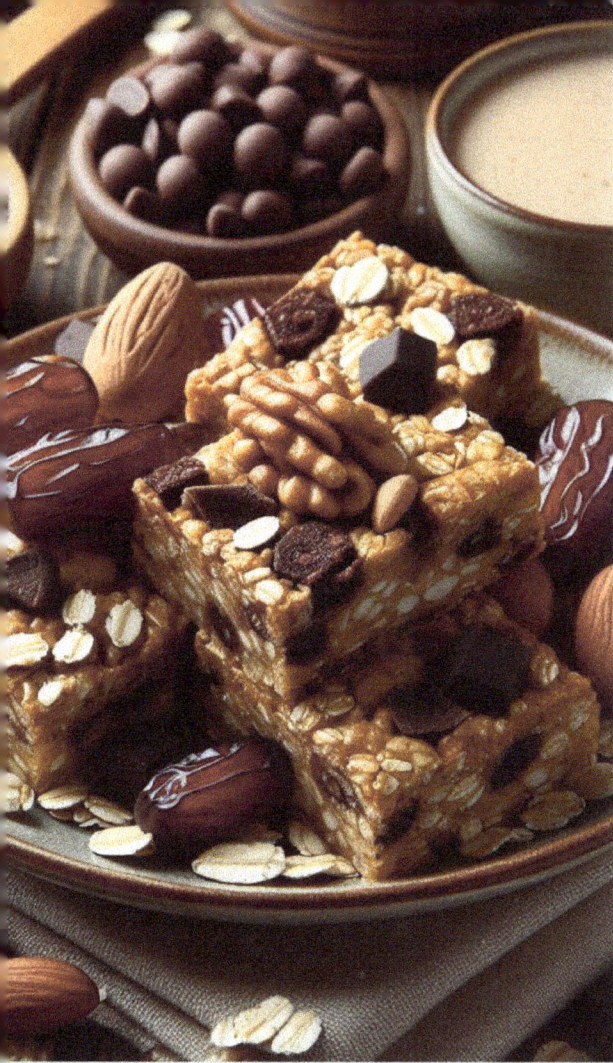

DATE AND NUT BREAKFAST BARS

Can be customized by adding your favourite nuts, seeds or dried fruits.

PREP TIME	FRIDGE TIME	SERVINGS
15 MINS	**1 HR**	**8-10 BARS**

Instructions

1. In a food processor, blend the pitted dates until a sticky paste. Add mixed nuts to the food processor and pulse until they are coarsely chopped.
2. In a large mixing bowl, combine date paste, chopped nuts, oats, almond butter, honey (or maple syrup), and a pinch of salt. Mix well until evenly combined.
3. Line a baking dish (8x8 inches or similar) with parchment paper. Press the mixture firmly into a lined baking dish using the back of a spoon or your hands. If desired, sprinkle additional nuts or seeds on top for extra crunch.
4. Refrigerate the mixture for at least 1 hour to set. Once firm, remove from the refrigerator and cut into bars or squares. Store the bars in an airtight container in the refrigerator for up to a week.

Ingredients

- 1 cup pitted dates (10-12 dates approx.)
- 1 cup mixed nuts
- 1 cup old-fashioned oats
- 1/4 cup nut butter of choice
- 1/4 cup honey or maple syrup
- 1/4 cup chocolate chips
- A pinch of salt

Notes:
- Mustaḥab foods included: Dates, Nuts and Honey

ZA'TAR AND CHEESE FATAYER (PIES)

These savoury pies are a delicious and filling breakfast option for Shahr Ramadan.

PREP TIME
2 HRS 15 MINS

COOK TIME
15 MINS

SERVINGS
8 PIES

Instructions

1. Preheat the oven to 350 F.
2. In a small bowl, combine lukewarm water, sugar, and yeast. Let it sit for about 10 minutes until frothy. In a large mixing bowl, combine flour, salt, and 2 tbsp olive oil. Add the yeast mixture and knead until you have a smooth dough. Cover and let it rise for about 2 hours until doubled in size.
3. Mix the za'atar spice with the crumbled feta cheese and 2 tbsp olive oil to create a flavorful paste.
4. Roll out dough into small circles (5 inches in diameter). Spread a generous amount of the za'atar cheese mixture onto each circle. Fold the dough to form a triangle shape and pinch the edges to seal. Arrange the fatayer on a baking sheet.
5. Bake for about 15 minutes or until golden brown.

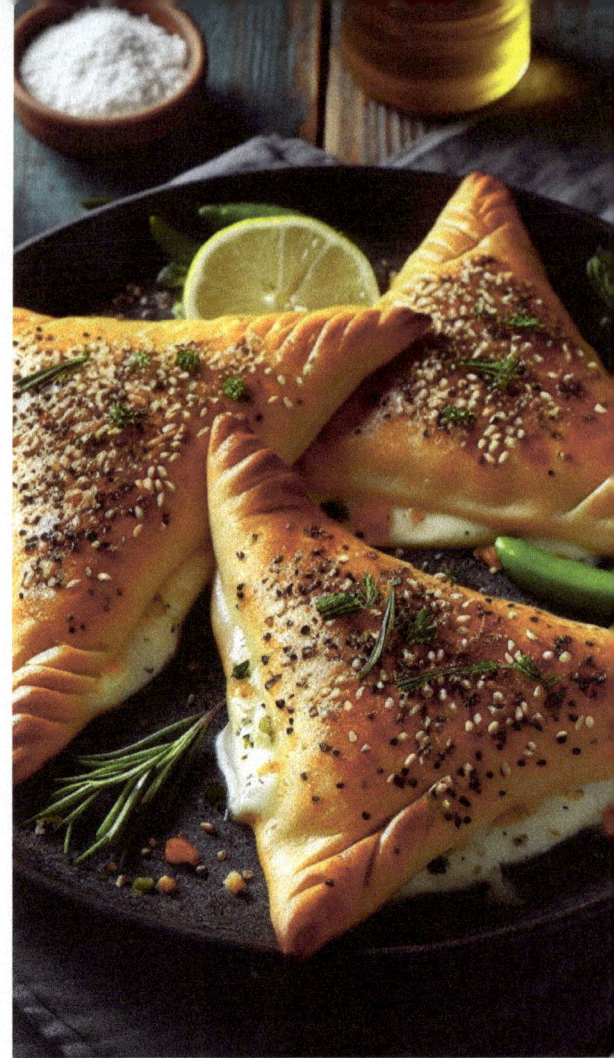

Ingredients

- 1 cup lukewarm water
- ½ tsp sugar
- 2 ¼ tsp active dry yeast (1 package)
- 3 cups unbleached all-purpose flour (plus more for dusting)
- 1 tsp salt
- 4 tbsp extra virgin olive oil
- ½ cup quality za'atar spice
- ½ cup crumbled feta cheese (or any mild cheese of your choice)

Notes:
- Mustaḥab foods included: cheese and olive oil

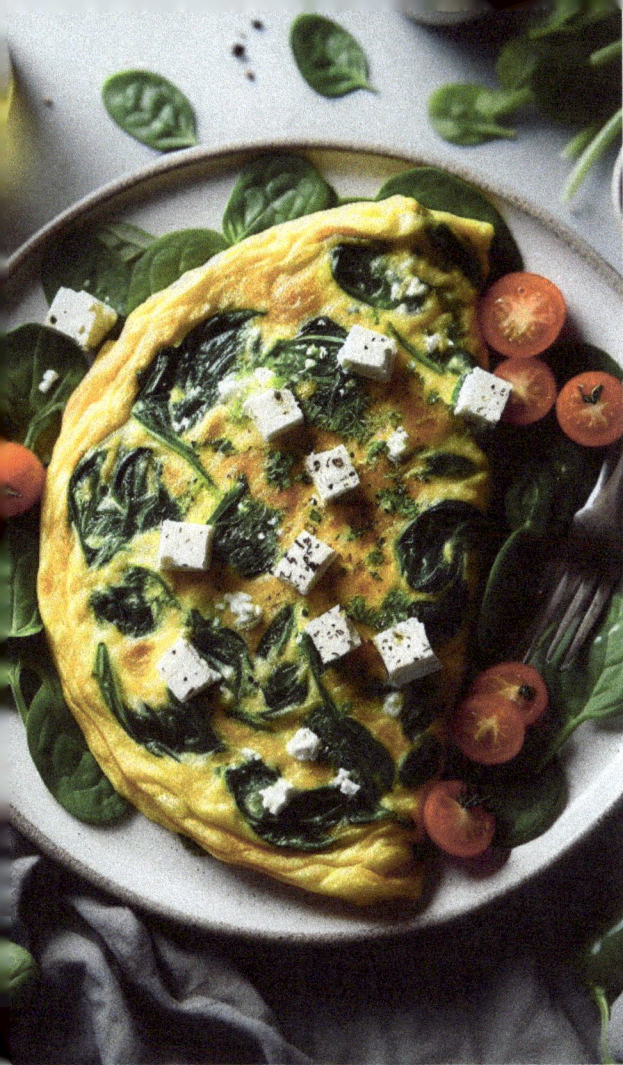

SPINACH AND FETA OMELETE

It's a perfect Suḥur meal, filled with protein and nutrients!

PREP TIME
2 MINS

COOK TIME
8 MINS

SERVINGS
1 PLATE

Instructions

1. Whisk the eggs in a small bowl and season with a pinch of salt and pepper.
2. Melt the butter in a small nonstick skillet over medium-low heat.
3. Add the baby spinach to the skillet and cook until wilted.
4. Pour the whisked eggs into the skillet, tilting it to coat the bottom evenly. Gently push the cooked eggs from the edges toward the center with a spatula, creating waves in the omelet.
5. Once the edges are set and the center is no longer runny, sprinkle the crumbled feta cheese over one-half of the omelet.
6. Fold the other half of the omelet over the cheese to create a half-moon shape. Slide the omelet onto a plate and serve immediately

Ingredients

- 2 large eggs
- A pinch of salt and pepper
- ½ tbsp unsalted butter
- 1 cup baby spinach
- 1/4 cup crumbled feta cheese

Notes:
- Mustaḥab foods included: Eggs and cheese.

TURKISH EGGS (ÇILBIR)

This famous Turkish dish combines the coolness of the garlicky yogurt with the richness of eggs, for a filling meal!

PREP TIME 3 MINS | **COOK TIME** 7 MINS | **SERVINGS** 1 PLATE

Instructions

1. To prepare the yogurt: In a bowl, whisk together the yogurt, minced garlic, and a pinch of salt. Divide this mixture between two serving bowls and set aside.
2. In a small pan, melt the butter or heat the olive oil. Add in half the paprika and mix until combined. Set aside.
3. In the same pan, fry the eggs to your liking, preferably as sunny side up.
4. To assemble: Spread a spoonful of the yogurt mix on the base of each serving bowl. Top with the eggs. Drizzle with the oil/butter sauce. Garnish with the parsley.
5. Serve with bread!

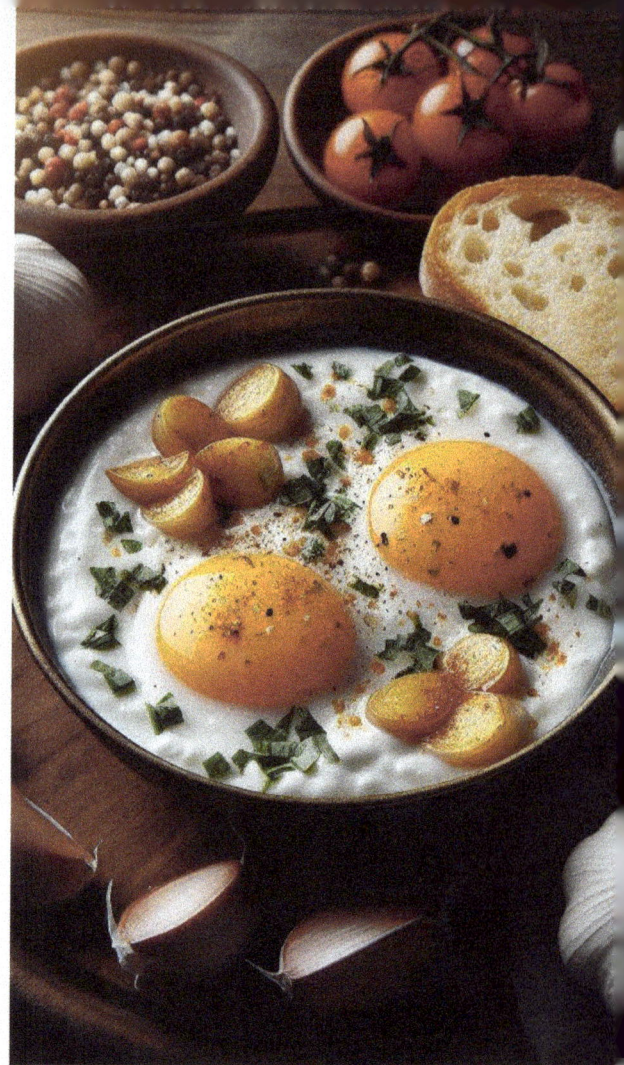

Ingredients

- 2 large eggs
- 1 cup labneh or greek yogurt (at room temp)
- ½ tsp minced garlic
- Salt, to taste
- 2 tbsp olive oil or melted butter
- 1 tsp for paprika (a little for granish)
- Fresh or dried parsley (for garnish)
- Bread (for serving)

Notes:
- Mustaḥab foods included: Yogurt, eggs, garlic and bread.

31

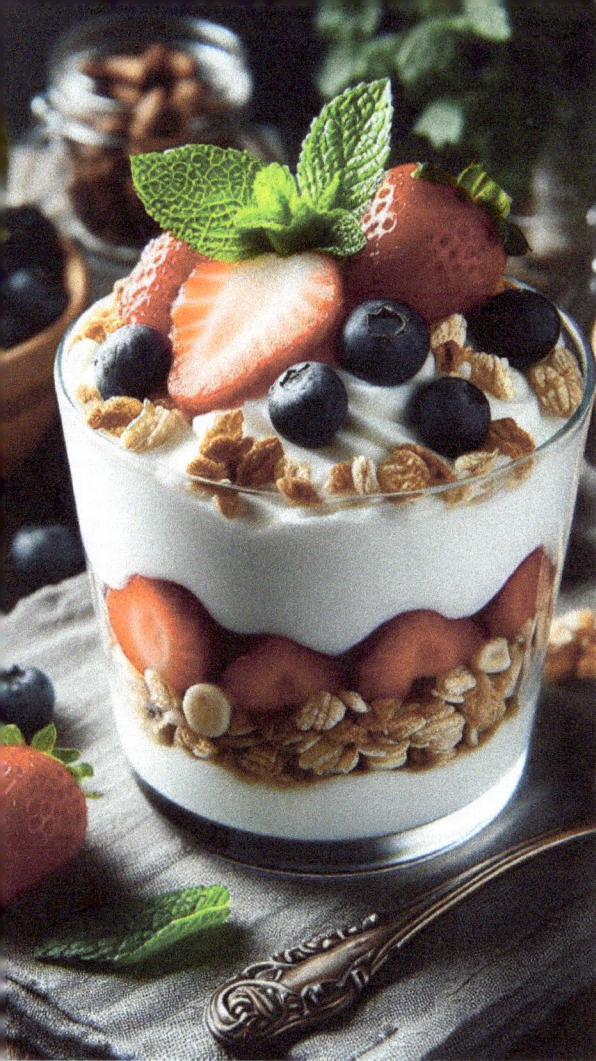

PARFAIT WITH MIXED BERRIES

This yogurt parfait is not only delicious but also packed with vitamins, fibre, and protein to keep you energized during your fast!

TOTAL TIME 10 MINS

SERVINGS 1 JAR

Instructions

1. In a glass or bowl, layer the ingredients as follows:
2. Start with about ¼ cup of yogurt (or half of a 5.5 oz container).
3. Add a layer of fresh berries (raspberries, strawberries, blueberries).
4. Sprinkle with granola.
5. Repeat the layers one more time.
6. Drizzle with maple syrup if desired.
7. Serve immediately and enjoy!

Notes:
- Mustaḥab foods included: yogurt and fruits.
- This recipe can be adjusted and recreated with any other fruits of your choice.

Ingredients

- 1 cup yogurt (fruit yogurt or unsweetened)
- ¾ cup fresh berries (raspberries, strawberries, blueberries)
- ⅓ cup granola
- 1 tsp maple syrup (optional, for added sweetness)

32

FRUIT SMOOTHIE BOWL

This smoothie bowl is packed with nutrients, protein, healthy fats and fibre.

TOTAL TIME
5 MINS

SERVINGS
1 BOWL

Instructions

1. In a blender, combine the frozen mango chunks, berries, banana, Greek yogurt, chia seeds, and milk.
2. Blend until you achieve a thick and creamy consistency. Adjust the coconut milk to reach your desired thickness.
3. Pour the smoothie into a bowl. Top with a topping of your choice and decorate! Topping options could be shredded coconut, sliced almonds or chocolate chips!

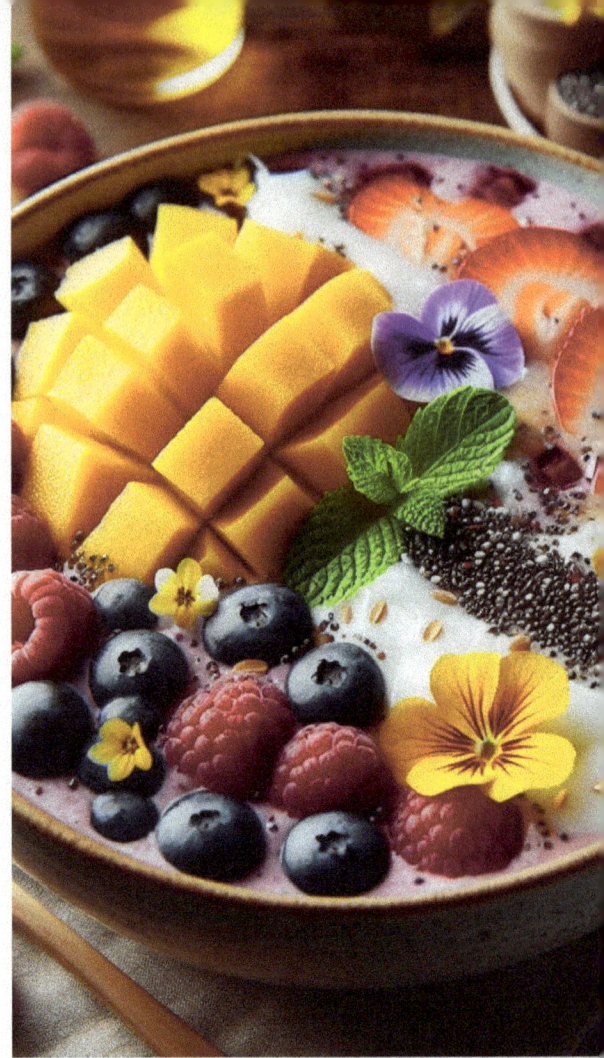

Notes:
- Mustaḥab foods included: fruits, yogurt and milk
- Topping options could be shredded coconut, sliced almonds or chocolate chips!

Ingredients

- ½ cup frozen mango chunks
- ½ cup frozen mixed berries (blueberries, strawberries)
- 1 small frozen ripe banana, frozen
- ¾ cup Greek yogurt
- 1 tbsp chia seeds
- ¼ cup coconut milk or milk of choice (adjustable)

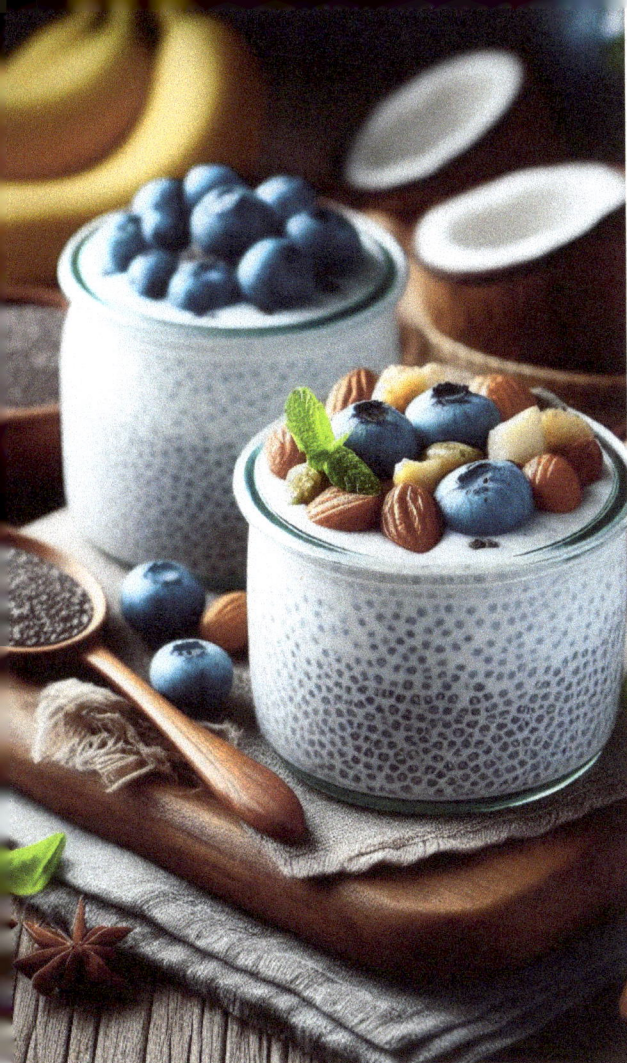

OVERNIGHT CHIA SEED PUDDING

This recipe is quick and can be prepared from the night before!

TOTAL TIME
5 MINS

SERVINGS
8 PIES

Instructions

1. Mix chia seeds and milk in a jar or bowl.
2. Add honey or maple syrup for sweetness.
3. Cover and refrigerate overnight.
4. In the morning, top with fresh fruits and your favourite toppings.

Ingredients

- 3 tbsp chia seeds
- 1 cup milk (or alternative like unsweeteened coconut milk)
- 1 tbsp honey or maple syrup
- Fresh fruits (such as berries or sliced banana)

Notes:
- Mustaḥab foods included: Milk, honey and fruits
- Optional toppings: nuts, shredded coconut, or granola
- This recipe can be adjusted to your liking, with combinations of fruits, nuts and seeds.

CHEESY CHICKPEA OMELET

Full of protein, healthy fat, fibre and other nutrients, this dish is sure to keep you satiated for a long day of fasting!

PREP TIME 3 MINS **COOK TIME** 7 MINS **SERVINGS** 1 PLATE

Instructions

1. In a bowl, whisk together chickpea flour, baking powder, salt, and black pepper.
2. Gradually add water, whisking until you have a smooth batter.
3. Heat olive oil in a non-stick skillet over medium heat.
4. Pour half of the batter into the skillet, spreading it evenly. Cook for 2-3 minutes until set and lightly golden.
5. Sprinkle half of the shredded cheese on one-half of the omelet.
6. Fold the omelet in half and cook for another minute. Repeat with the remaining batter and cheese.
7. Serve hot, garnished with fresh parsley or chives.

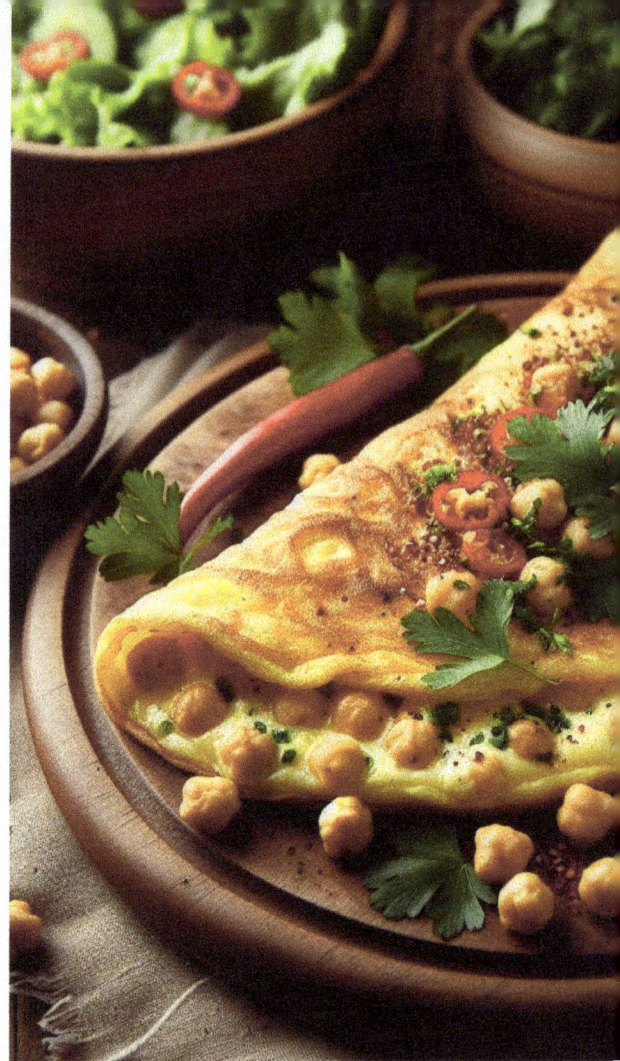

Ingredients

- 1 cup chickpea flour
- 1 tsp baking powder
- Salt and black pepper, to taste
- ½ cup water
- ½ cup shredded cheese of choice
- 1 tbsp olive oil
- Fresh parsley or chives, chopped (for garnish)

Notes:
- Mustaḥab foods included: chickpea and olive oil

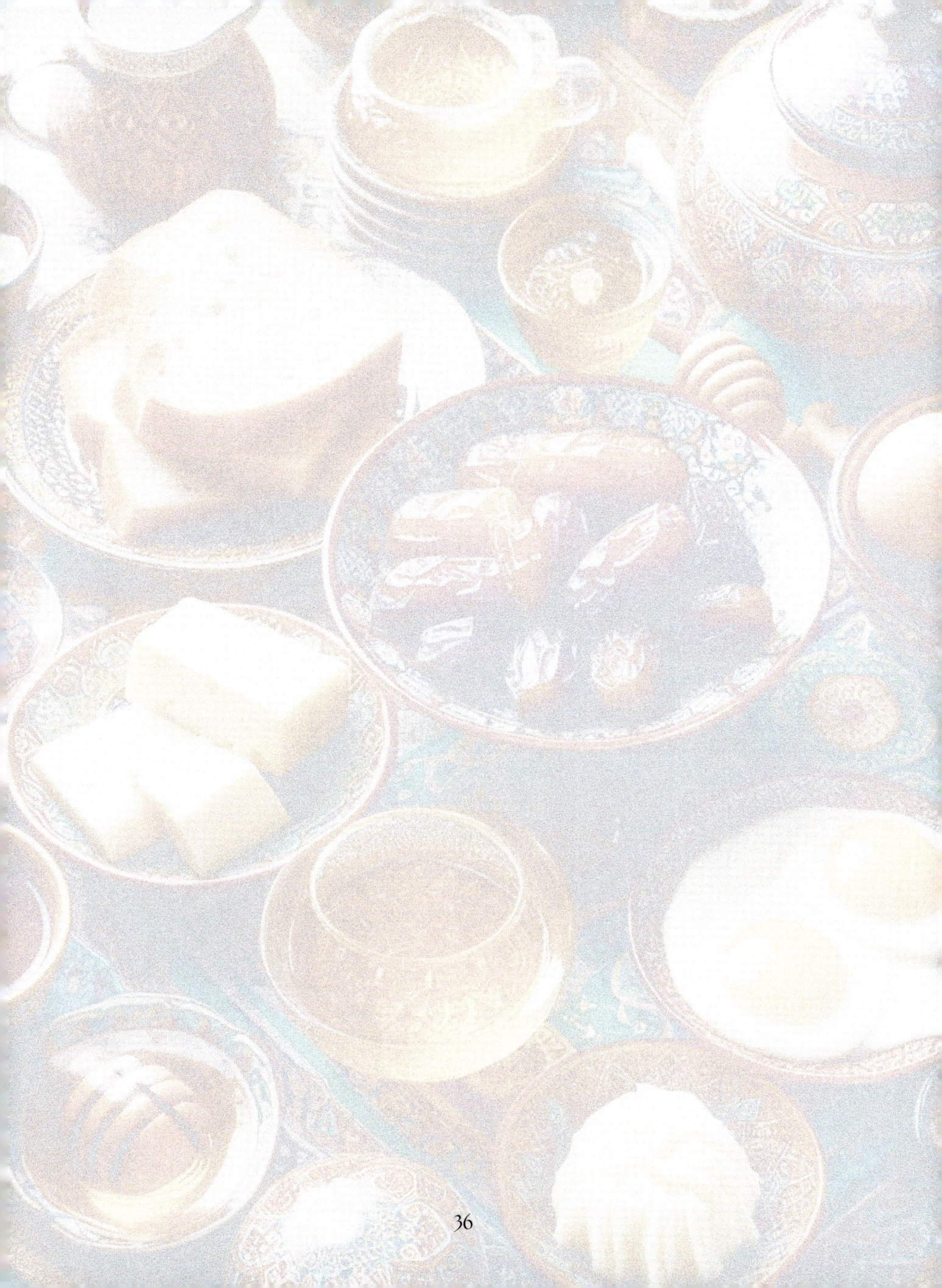

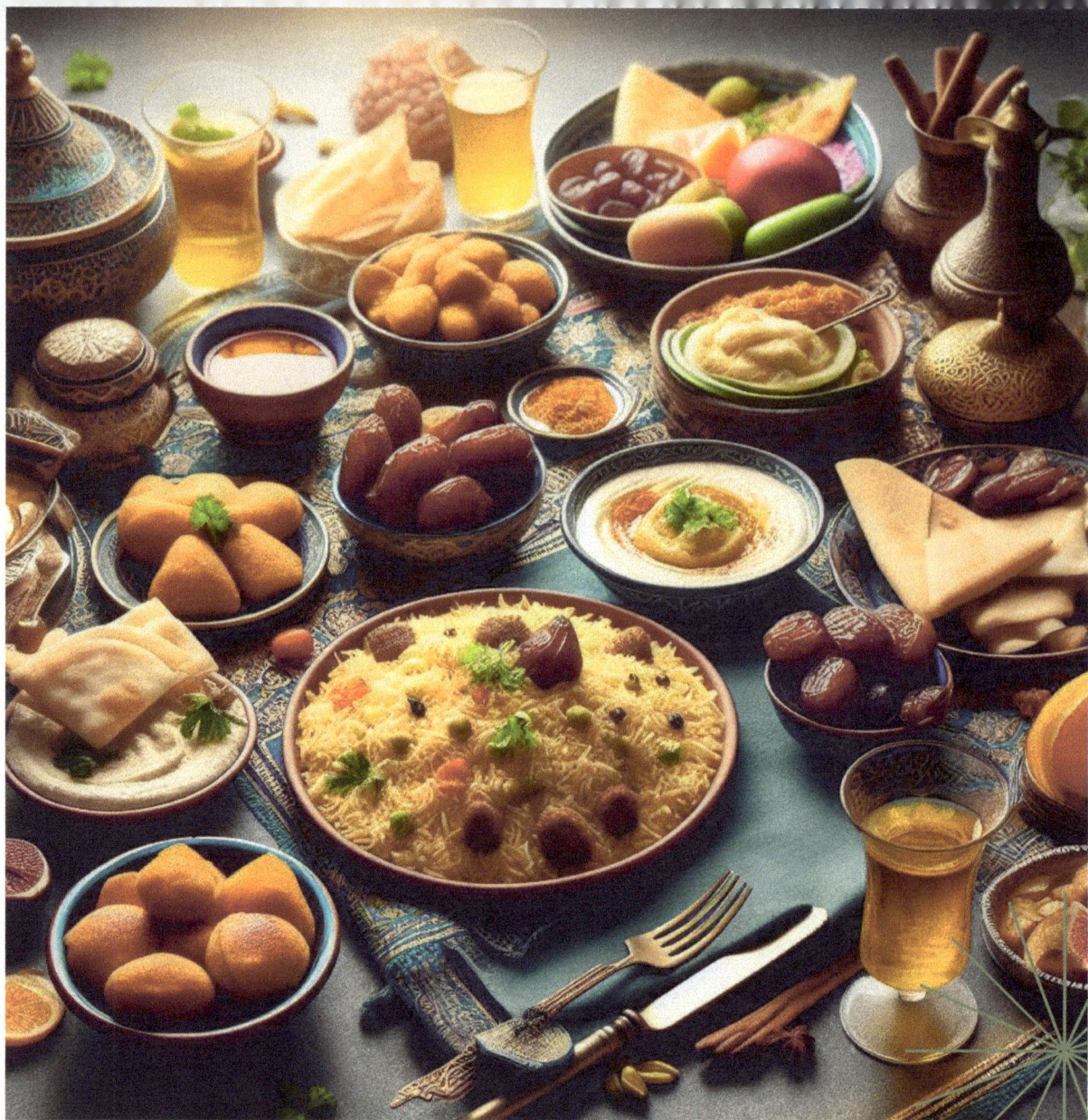

breaking of the fast

Ifṭār

IFTĀR : BREAKING OF THE FAST

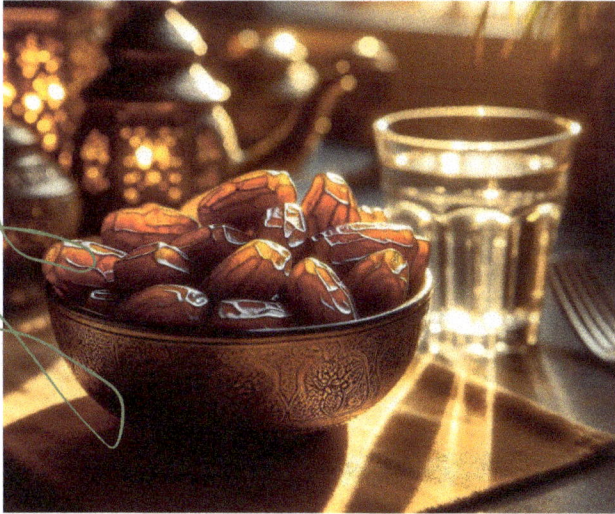

History states that on the first day of fasting, Imam al-Sajjād (as) would ensure sharing a meal with others. It was his honourable tradition to prepare food and distribute it to various families in his city. This act exemplifies compassion and generosity, especially in this month. It is important to remember that Iftār is also about connecting with the community and remembering to practice gratitude.

The Ma'ṣūmīn (as) have highlighted that breaking one's fast with a Ḥalāl means doubling the reward of the prayer to four hundredfold.

There are various recommendations for Iftār – breaking of one's fast. The Ahlulbayt (as) have encouraged starting with warm water, milk, ripe dates or fruits [1]. These foods replenish the body's energy and nutrient stores by providing crucial vitamins and minerals. They further support easing the transition from fasting to eating.

The Imam (as) said, "A fasting person has two sources of joy: when he breaks his fast and at meeting his Lord. [2]"

Imam al-Ṣādiq (as) also said that breaking the fast with a bit of warm water nourishes the body, cleanses the liver, washes away sins from the heart, and strengthens one's eyesight and pupils [3].

It is also mentioned that starting with a piece of candy (or sweet) is beneficial. Shaykh al-Mufīd stated that it is also permissible to eat a piece of the soil of Imam al-Ḥusayn (as)'s grave, as it is a cure [4].

1] Wasā`il al-Shia
2] al-Kāfī, Vol. 4, Pg. 65, Ḥadīth 15
3] al-Kāfī, Vol. 4, Chp. 66, Ḥadīth 2
4] Mafātīḥ al-Jinān

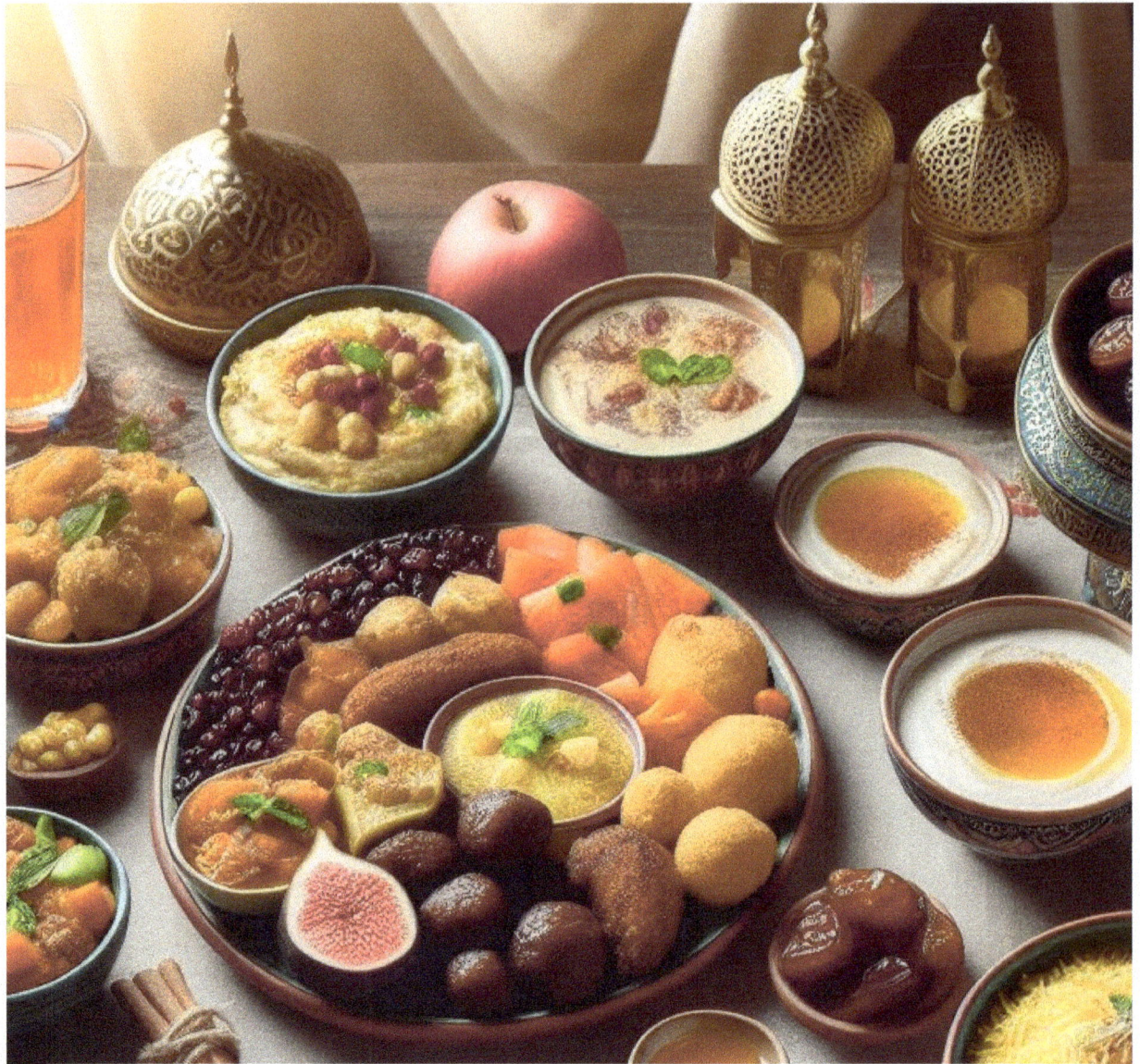

IFṬĀR

Types of food to include for Ifṭār

LENTILS

According to Imam Ali (as), eating lentils softens the heart and increases tears. The A`immah (as) has also recommended eating lentil-based porridge/stew as it takes away thirst (especially for a long day of fasting), provides energy, cures illnesses and has a cooling effect on the stomach.

These benefits are backed by science. This humble legume is a plant-based protein, supports cardiovascular health, is a complex carbohydrate, contains antioxidant properties and is rich in nutrients [3].

1] al-Kāfī, Vol. 6, Bk. 5, Chp. 93, Ḥadīth 1
2] al-Kāfī, Vol. 6, Bk. 5, Chp. 54, Ḥadīth 1
3] McQueen, J. (2022, August 15). Health benefits of legumes. WebMD. https://www.webmd.com/food-recipes/health-benefits-legumes

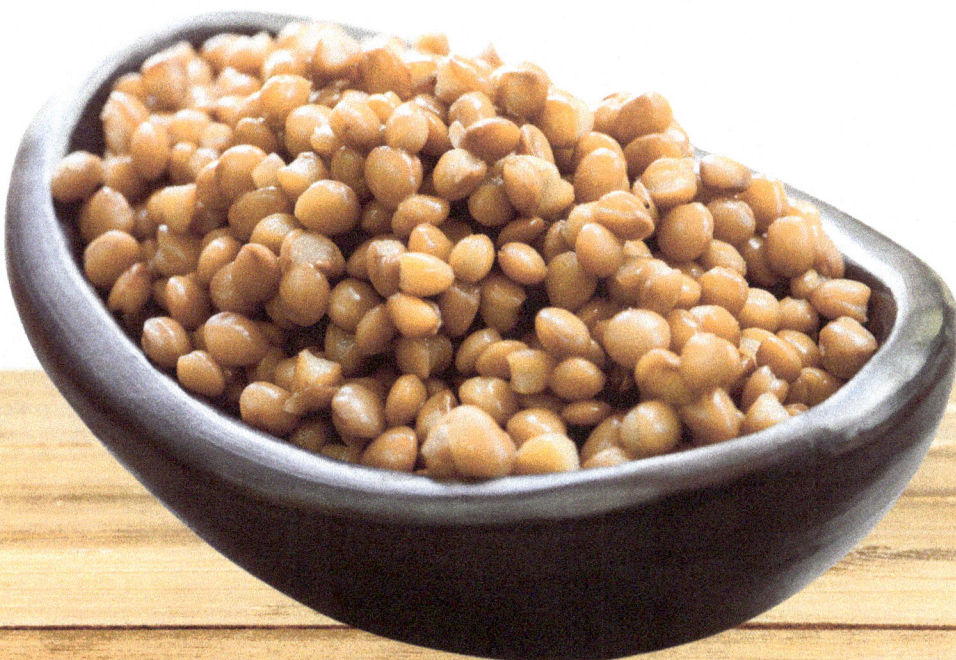

BARLEY

The Ma'ṣūmīn (as) have emphasized the excellence of barley, specifically barley bread by stating it is the food of the prophets and removes illnesses [1].

Barley is a versatile whole grain, rich in vitamins and minerals like manganese, iron, thiamine and vitamin B6. It is high in fibre, supports heart health, improves digestion and has antioxidant properties shown to reduce the risk of cancer and heart disease [2]. It is gentle on the stomach yet filling after a long day of fasting!

1] [al-Kāfī, Vol. 6, Bk. 5, Chp. 51, Ḥadīth 1]
2] Evans, C. E. L. (2019). Dietary fibre and cardiovascular health: a review of current evidence and policy. Proceedings of the Nutrition Society, 79(1), 61–67. https://doi.org/10.1017/s0029665119000673

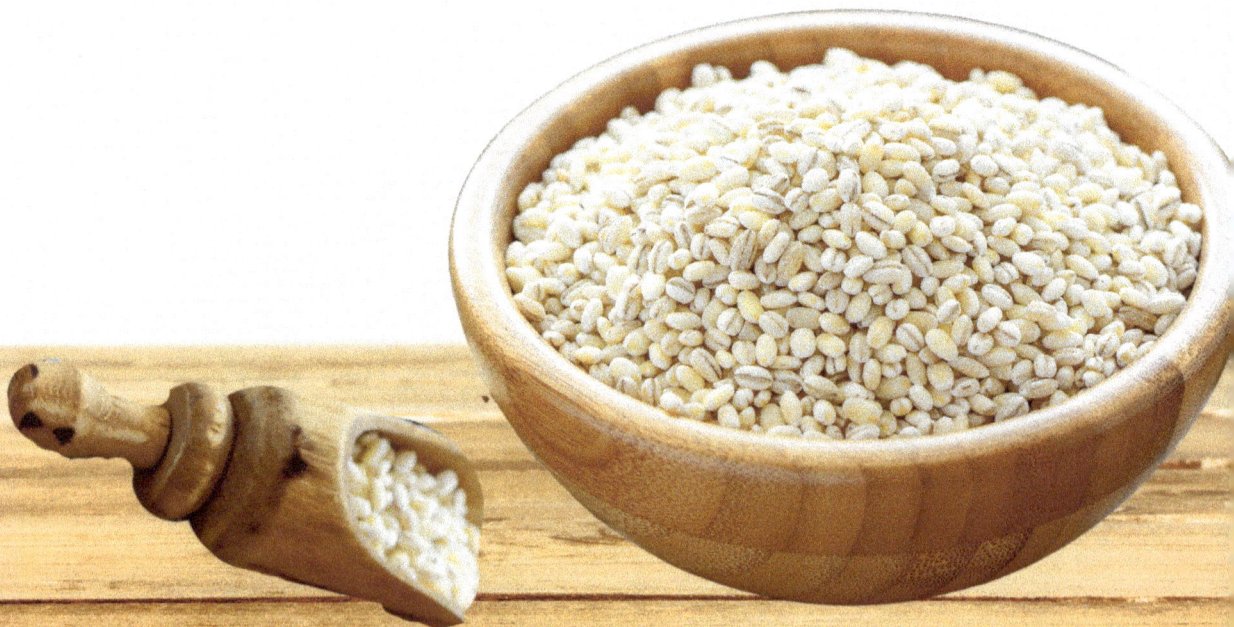

RICE

The Holy A`immah (as) have spoken of rice being advantageous for gut health and in reducing hemorrhoids [1].

Rice is rich in carbohydrates, which can replenish one's energy after fasting. It is low in fat and sodium and contains various vitamins and minerals. Brown rice is a healthy option, containing fibre which is nutrient-dense and beneficial for intestinal health [2].

1] al-Kāfī, Vol. 6, Bk. 5, Chp. 91, Ḥadīth 2]
2] Pandey, S., K.R. Lijini, & A. Jayadeep. (2017). Medicinal and Health Benefits of Brown Rice. Springer Nature. https://doi.org/10.1007/978-3-319-59011-0_7

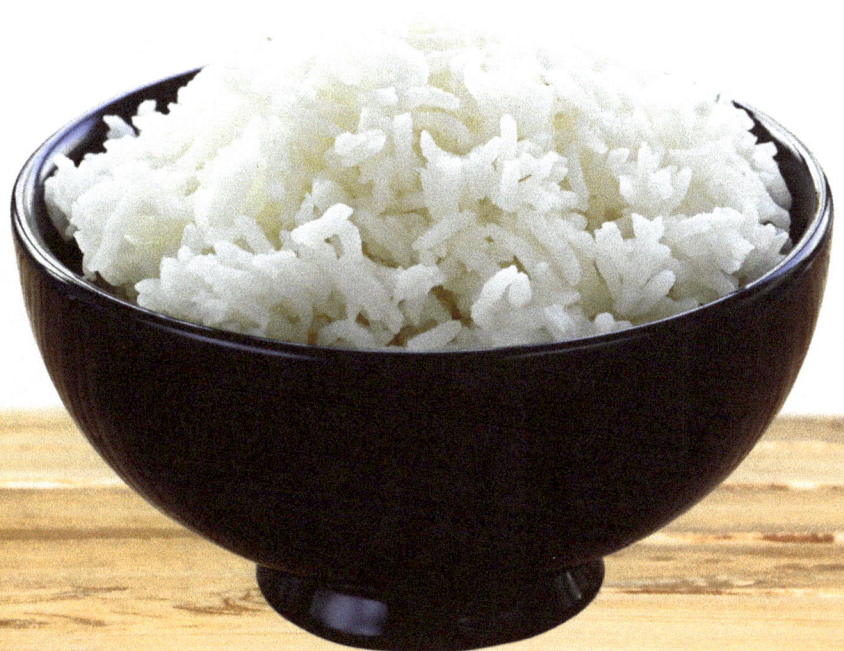

BEANS

The 6th Imam (as) said about the following beans: eating fava cleanses the stomach, kidney beans help dispel gases [1] and chickpeas are good for back pain [2].

Beans are complex carbohydrates, rich in protein, high in fibre and contain vitamins and minerals like folate, iron and potassium [3]. This makes them a great choice for an Iftār meal as they can provide quick energy.

1] al-Kāfī, Vol. 6, Bk. 5, Chp. 94, Ḥadīth 4
2] al-Kāfī, Vol. 6, Bk. 5, Chp. 92, Ḥadīth 4
3] Rebello, C. J., Greenway, F. L., & Finley, J. W. (2014). A review of the nutritional value of legumes and their effects on obesity and its related co-morbidities. Obesity Reviews, 15(5), 392–407. https://doi.org/10.1111/obr.12144

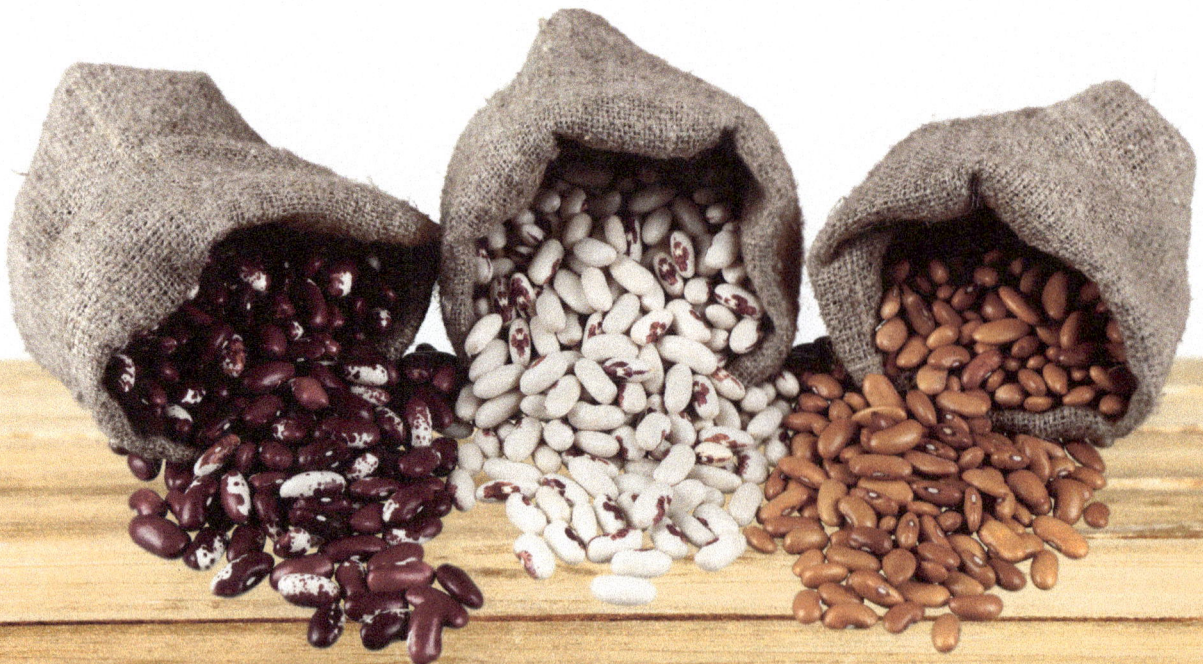

OTHER MUSTAHAB FOODS
perfect for Iftār

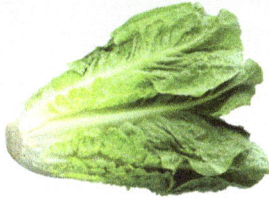

lettuce [1]

Full of fibre, essential nutrients and has a high water content

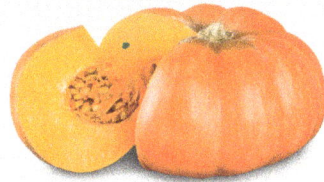

pumpkin [2]

provides energy, aids digestion and is a source of vit. A & C

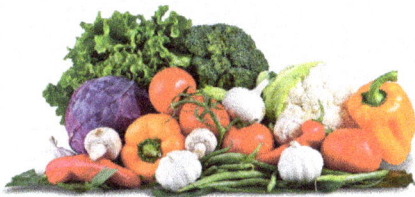

vegetables [3]

offers vitamins, minerals and supports health

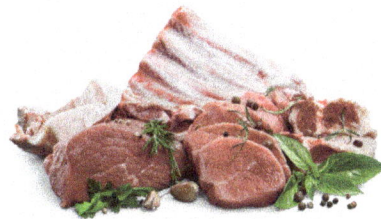

meat [4]

Supports muscle health, rich in protein, iron and B vitamins.

Combining these foods will create a well-balanced and nourishing Iftār!

1] Al-Kāfī, Vol. 6, Bk. 5, Chp. 118, Ḥadith 1
2] Al-Maḥāsin, Vol. 2, Bk. 3, Ḥadith 729
3] Al-Kāfī, Vol. 6, Bk. 5
4] Al-Kāfī, Vol. 6, Bk. 5, Chp. 55

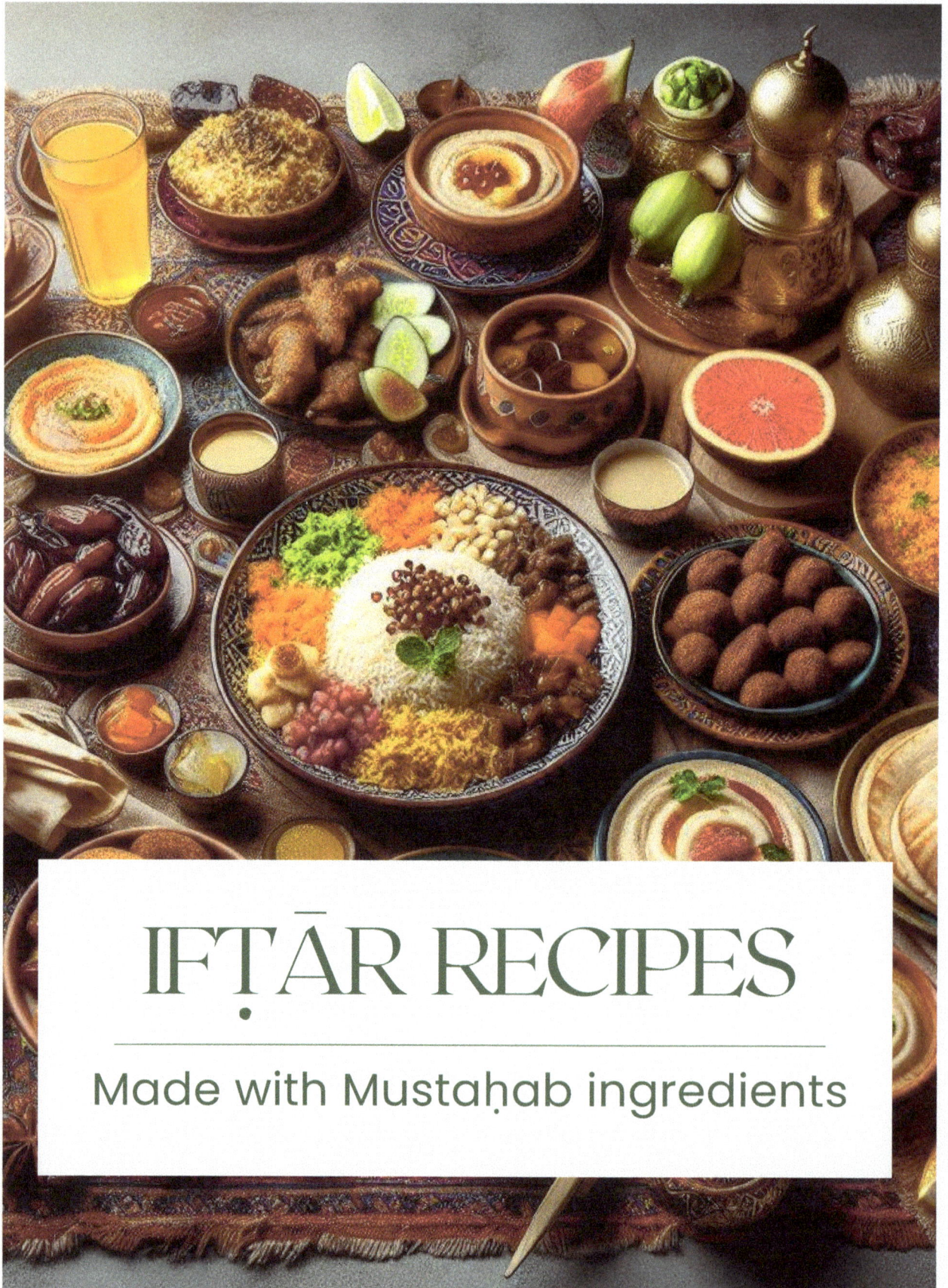

IFṬĀR RECIPES

Made with Mustaḥab ingredients

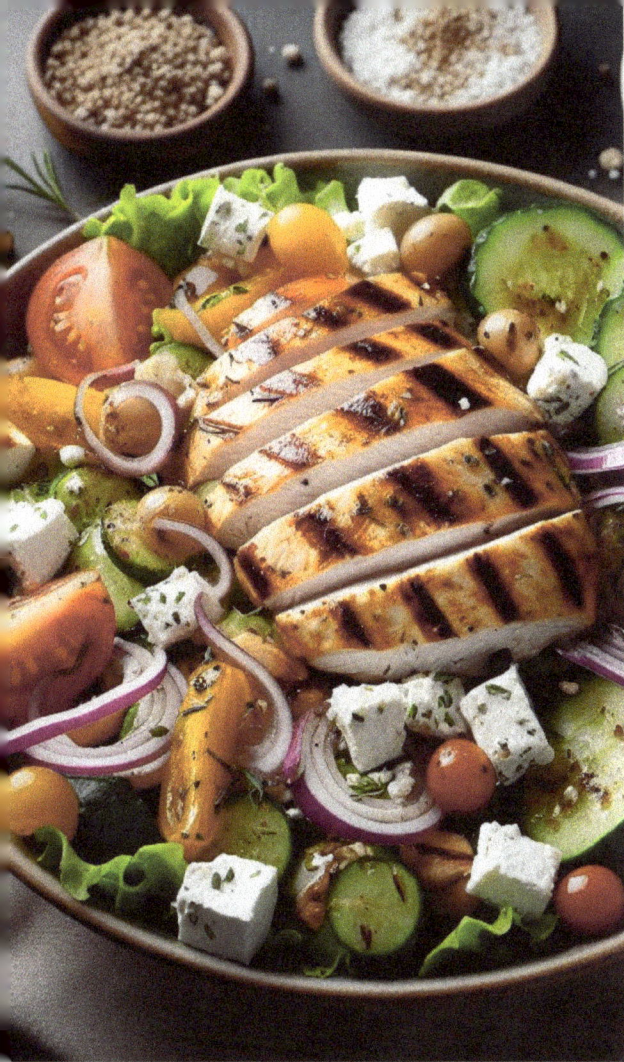

GRILLED CHICKEN SALAD

This refreshing salad is hydrating and filling, perfect as an iftar appetizer!

PREP TIME 20 MINS

COOK TIME 10 MINS

SERVINGS 2-3

Instructions

1. Grill chicken breast until fully cooked. Season with salt, pepper, and a touch of olive oil for extra flavour. Once done, slice into thin strips.
2. Tear mixed greens into bite-sized pieces and place them in a large salad bowl. Combine cherry tomatoes, cucumber, onions and bell peppers.
3. Assemble: Add grilled chicken slices on top of the salad greens. Add cherry tomatoes, cucumber, red onion, and bell peppers over the chicken. Drizzle extra virgin olive oil over the salad. Squeeze fresh lemon juice, and season with salt and pepper according to your taste. Crumble feta cheese (optional). Toss, all the ingredients together to ensure they are well combined. Serve Immediately.

Notes:
- Mustaḥab foods included: cucumber, lettuce and onion

Ingredients

- 2 chicken breasts, grilled and sliced.
- 4 cups Mixed salad greens (lettuce, spinach etc.)
- Around 1 cup cherry tomatoes:, halved.
- 1 medium cucumber, peeled and diced.
- ½ red onion, thinly sliced.
- 1 cup of sliced bell peppers.
- Olive oil (drizzle as needed)
- Juice of 1 lemon.
- Salt and pepper to taste
- Feta Cheese (optional)

OTTOMAN STYLE LENTIL SOUP

This soup is comforting, nutritious, light on the stomach and filling!

PREP TIME
10 MINS

COOK TIME
10 MINS

SERVINGS
1 PLATE

Instructions

1. In a large pot, sauté the chopped onion and minced garlic in a little olive oil until softened.
2. Add the diced carrot and chopped celery, and cook for a few minutes.
3. Add the rinsed lentils, vegetable or chicken broth, ground cumin, and ground turmeric.
4. Bring the mixture to a boil, then reduce the heat and simmer for about 20-25 minutes, or until the lentils are tender.
5. Season with salt and pepper to taste. Use an immersion blender or a regular blender to puree the soup until smooth (optional).
6. Stir in the lemon juice.
7. Serve hot, garnished with fresh parsley or cilantro.

Notes:
- Mustaḥab foods included: lentils, onions, garlic, celery, carrot and lemon.

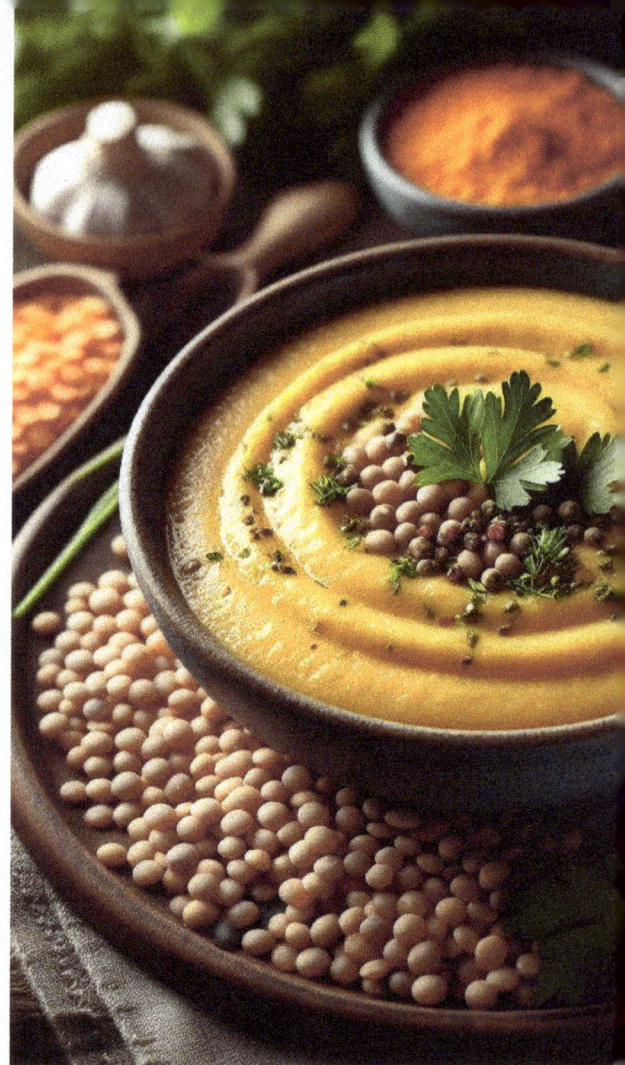

Ingredients

- 1 cup red lentils (rinsed and drained)
- 1 onion, chopped
- 2 cloves of garlic, minced
- 1 carrot, peeled and diced
- 1 celery stalk, chopped
- 4 cups vegetable or chicken broth
- 1 tsp ground cumin
- 1 tsp ground turmeric
- Salt and pepper to taste
- Juice of half a lemon
- Fresh parsley or cilantro for garnish

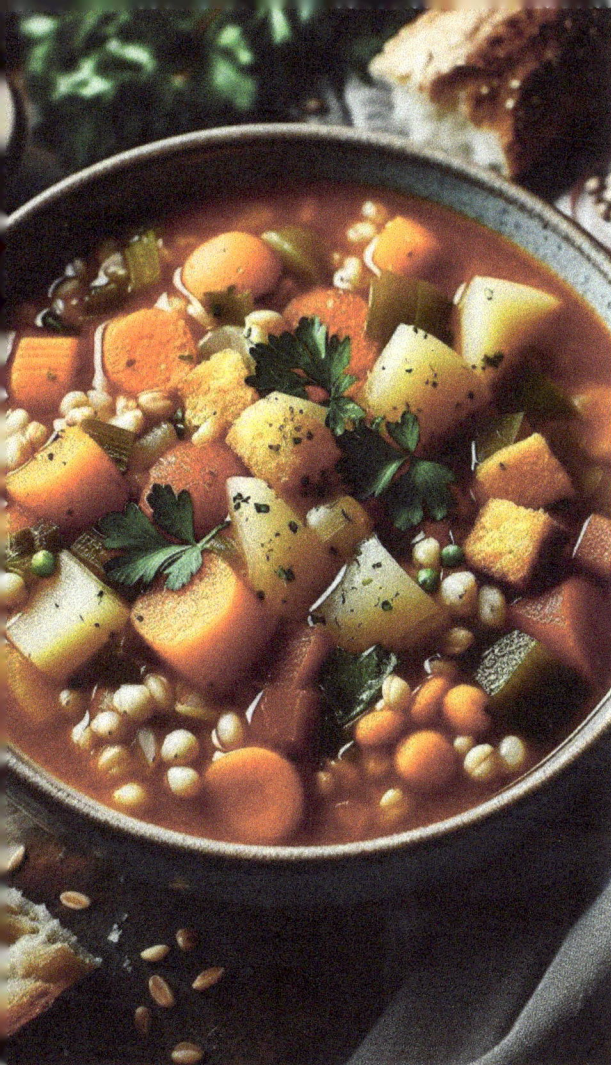

HEARTY BARLEY VEGETABLE STEW

Stews are always a go-to in this month! This one is rich in fibre, vitamins and minerals!

PREP TIME 10 MINS   **COOK TIME** 40 MINS   **SERVINGS** 2-3

Instructions

1. In a large pot, sauté the chopped onion and minced garlic in a little olive oil until softened.
2. Add the diced carrots, chopped celery, and zucchini. Cook for a few minutes.
3. Add the rinsed barley, vegetable or chicken broth, ground cumin, and ground coriander.
4. Bring the mixture to a boil, then reduce the heat and simmer for about 30–40 minutes, or until the barley is tender.
5. Season with salt and pepper to taste. Serve hot, garnished with fresh parsley.

Notes:
- Mustaḥab foods included: barley, onion, garlic and carrots.

Ingredients

- 1 cup barley (rinsed and drained)
- 1 onion, chopped
- 2 cloves of garlic, minced
- 2 carrots, peeled and diced
- 2 celery stalks, chopped
- 1 zucchini, diced
- 4 cups vegetable or chicken broth
- 1 tsp ground cumin
- 1 tsp ground coriander
- Salt and pepper to taste
- Fresh parsley for garnish

CHICKEN AND RICE ONE-TRAY BAKE

Baked to perfection, it's a comforting and flavourful meal that's quick to make!

PREP TIME
7 MINS

COOK TIME
35 MINS

SERVINGS
4-6

Instructions

1. Preheat your oven to 375ºF (190ºC).
2. In an oven-safe dish, layer the sliced onion, minced garlic, and chicken thighs.
3. Sprinkle the ground spices (cinnamon, black pepper, salt) over the chicken.
4. Rinse the rice and spread it evenly over the chicken.
5. Pour the chicken broth over everything.
6. Cover the dish with foil or a lid. Bake for about 30 minutes or until the chicken is cooked and the rice is tender.
7. Garnish with chopped parsley before serving.

Ingredients

- 1 lb boneless, skinless chicken thighs
- 1 cup basmati rice
- 1 onion, thinly sliced
- 2 cloves garlic, minced
- 1 tsp ground cinnamon
- 1 tsp ground black pepper
- 1 tsp salt
- 2 cups chicken broth
- Chopped fresh parsley for garnish

Notes:
- Mustaḥab foods included: rice and garlic.

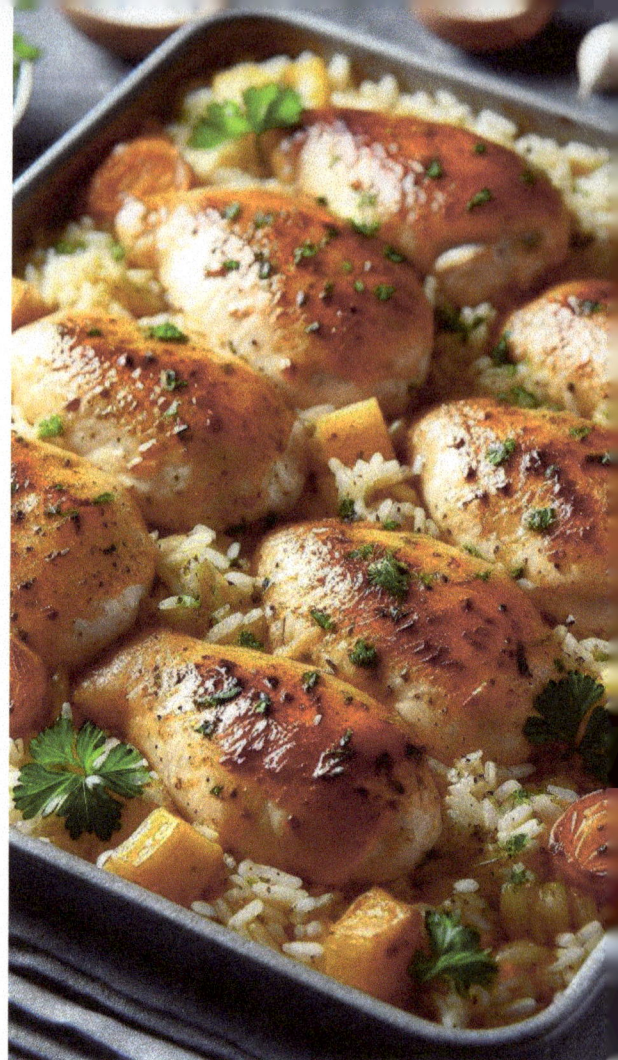

49

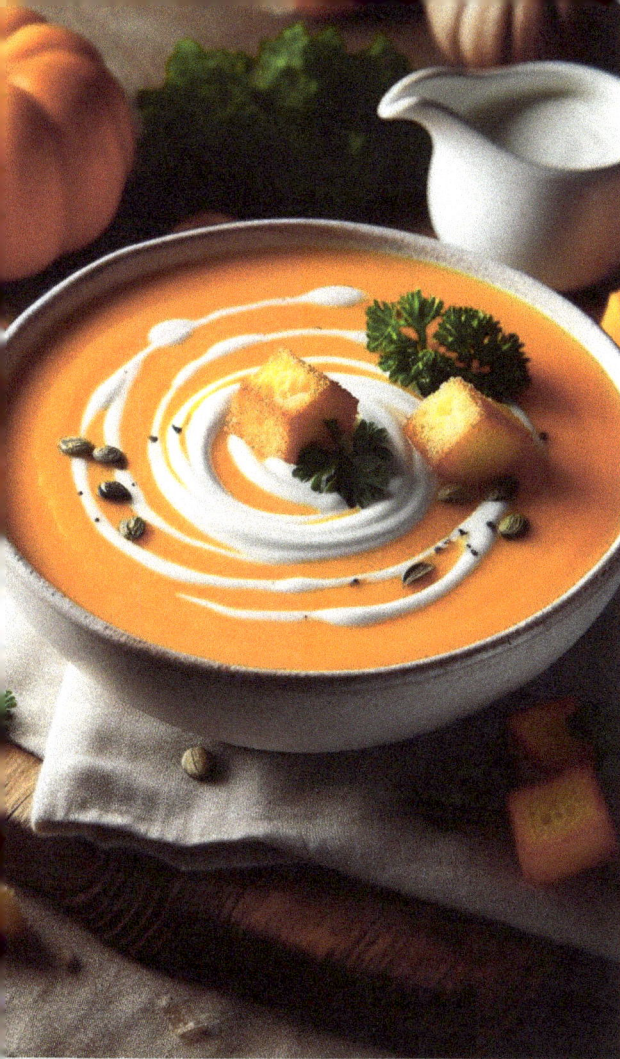

CARROT PUMPKIN SOUP

This warm soup is easy on the stomach and highly nutritious!

PREP TIME 10 MINS | **COOK TIME** 40 MINS | **SERVINGS** 2-3

Instructions

1. Heat olive oil in a saucepan (or 4-quart Dutch oven) over medium heat. Add chopped onion and minced garlic. Sauté for 2 to 3 minutes until soft and translucent.
2. Add cubed pumpkin, sliced carrots, ground cumin, ground coriander, salt, and black pepper. Cook for another 5 minutes, stirring occasionally.
3. Pour in the vegetable or chicken stock. Bring to a simmer and cover the pot.
4. Let the soup simmer for about 20-25 minutes or until the pumpkin and carrots are tender.
5. Use an immersion blender to puree the soup. Taste and adjust seasoning if needed.
6. Serve hot with optional toppings like toasted pumpkin seeds, fresh parsley, or a drizzle of cream.

Notes:
- Mustaḥab foods included: pumpkin, carrot, onion, garlic and olive oil.

Ingredients

- 1 tbsp olive oil
- 1 medium onion, chopped
- 1 ½ tbsp minced garlic
- 2 cups of frozen cubed pumpkin
- 2 large carrots, peeled and sliced
- 4 cups vegetable or chicken stock
- 1 tsp ground cumin
- ½ tsp ground coriander
- Salt and black pepper, to taste
- Optional toppings: toasted pumpkin seeds, fresh parsley, or a drizzle of cream

ARABIC BEAN STEW (FUSULIA YABSA)

This is an ideal iftār choice due to its sustaining energy, protein & fibre content, and essential nutrients!

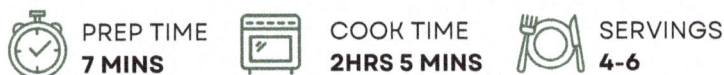

PREP TIME 7 MINS

COOK TIME 2HRS 5 MINS

SERVINGS 4-6

Instructions

1. In a large pot, heat some vegetable oil and sauté the chopped onion until translucent.
2. Add the minced garlic and cubed meat (if using). Brown the meat on all sides.
3. Stir in the tomato paste, ground cumin, ground coriander, salt, and pepper.
4. Add the soaked and drained white beans to the pot.
5. Pour in enough water to cover the beans and meat (about 4 cups).
6. Bring to a boil, then reduce the heat and simmer, partially covered, for about 1.5 to 2 hours or until the beans are tender and the flavours meld.
7. Adjust the seasoning if needed. Serve hot over cooked rice.

Notes:
- Mustaḥab foods included: beans, meat, onion, garlic and rice

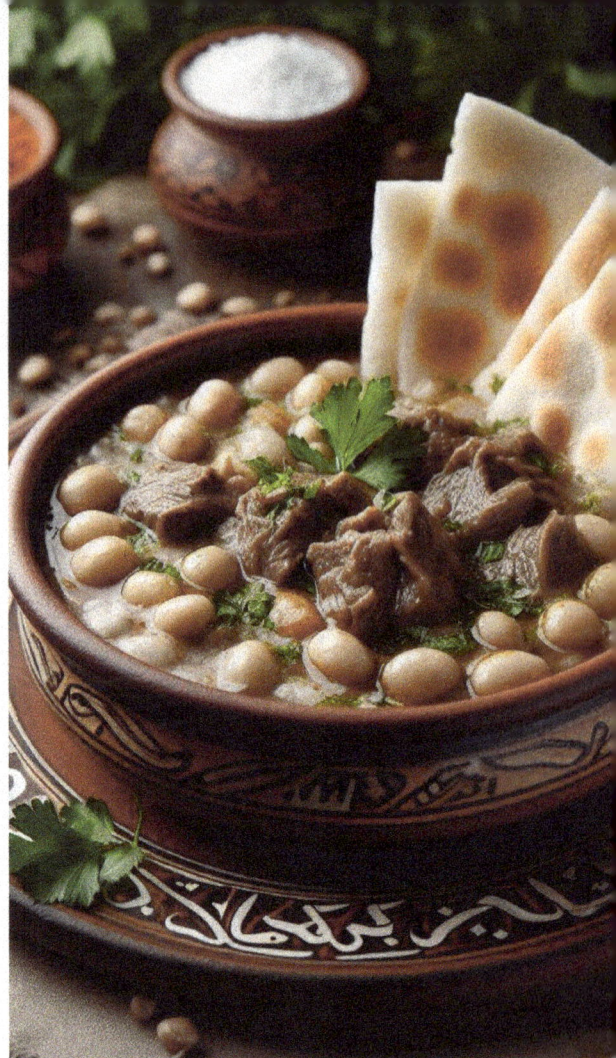

Ingredients

- 1 cup dried white beans (such as navy beans or cannellini beans), soaked overnight and drained
- 1 lb meat (lamb, beef, or chicken), cubed
- 1 large onion, finely chopped
- 3 cloves garlic, minced
- 2 tbsp tomato paste
- 1 tsp ground cumin
- 1 tsp ground coriander
- Salt and pepper, to taste
- Water (about 4 cups)
- Vegetable oil for sautéing
- Cooked rice (for serving)

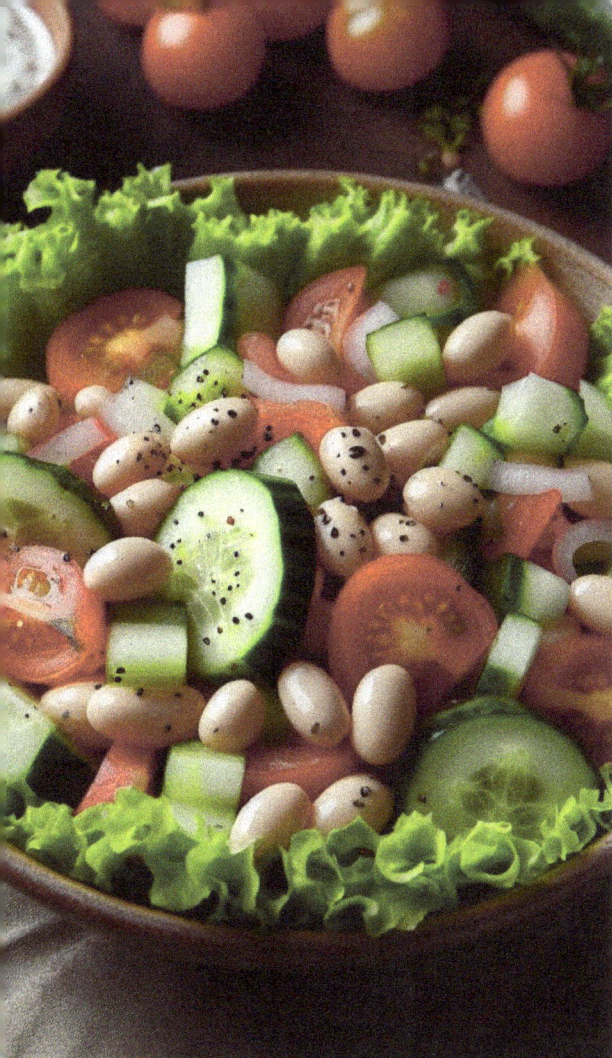

WHITE BEAN MIXED VEGETABLE SALAD

This refreshing salad is hydrating and filling, perfect as an iftār appetizer!

TOTAL TIME 15 MINS

SERVINGS 4

Instructions

1. In a large mixing bowl, combine the white beans, diced cucumber, diced tomatoes, and sliced red onion.
2. Add the torn lettuce leaves to the bowl.
3. Drizzle with olive oil and lime or lemon juice. Season with salt and black pepper.
4. Toss everything together until well combined.
5. Garnish with fresh parsley or dill. Serve chilled.

Ingredients

- 1 can (15 oz) white beans, drained and rinsed
- 1 large cucumber, diced
- 2 ripe tomatoes, diced
- ½ small red onion, thinly sliced
- 1 head of lettuce torn into bite-sized pieces
- Fresh parsley or dill, chopped
- Juice of 2-3 fresh limes or lemons
- Extra virgin olive oil
- Salt and black pepper, to taste

Notes:
- Mustaḥab foods included: beans, cucumber, onion, lettuce, lemon and olive oil

MEAT-STUFFED PUFF PASTRY

This side is a wonderful replacement for other unhealthier fried foods.

PREP TIME 5 MINS   **COOK TIME** 30-40 MINS   **SERVINGS** 4-6

Instructions

1. Preheat oven according to pastry package instructions.
2. In a skillet, cook ground meat over medium heat until browned. Drain excess fat. Add onion, garlic, ground cumin, coriander, salt, and black pepper to the skillet. Cook until the onion is soft and fragrant.
3. Roll out the puff pastry sheet on a floured surface. Cut into squares or rectangles (4x4 inches each). Place a spoonful of meat mixture in the center of each pastry square. Fold the pastry over the filling to create a triangle or rectangle shape. Press the edges to seal. Beat an egg and brush it over the top of each pastry for a golden finish.
4. Place the pastries on a parchment-lined baking sheet. Bake for 15-20 minutes or until puffed and golden.
5. Garnish with fresh parsley and serve warm.

Notes:
- Mustaḥab foods included: Meat and onion

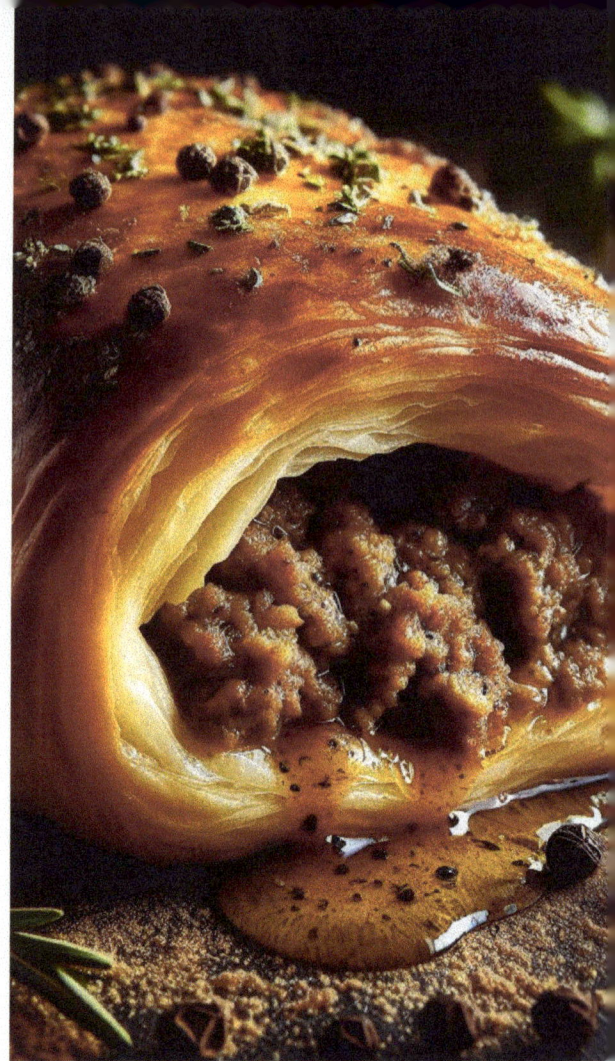

Ingredients

- 1 sheet of store-bought puff pastry (thawed if frozen)
- ½ pound ground beef or lamb
- 1 small onion, finely chopped
- 2 cloves garlic, minced
- 1 tsp ground cumin
- 1 tsp ground coriander
- Salt and black pepper, to taste
- Fresh parsley, chopped (for garnish)
- 1 egg (for egg wash)

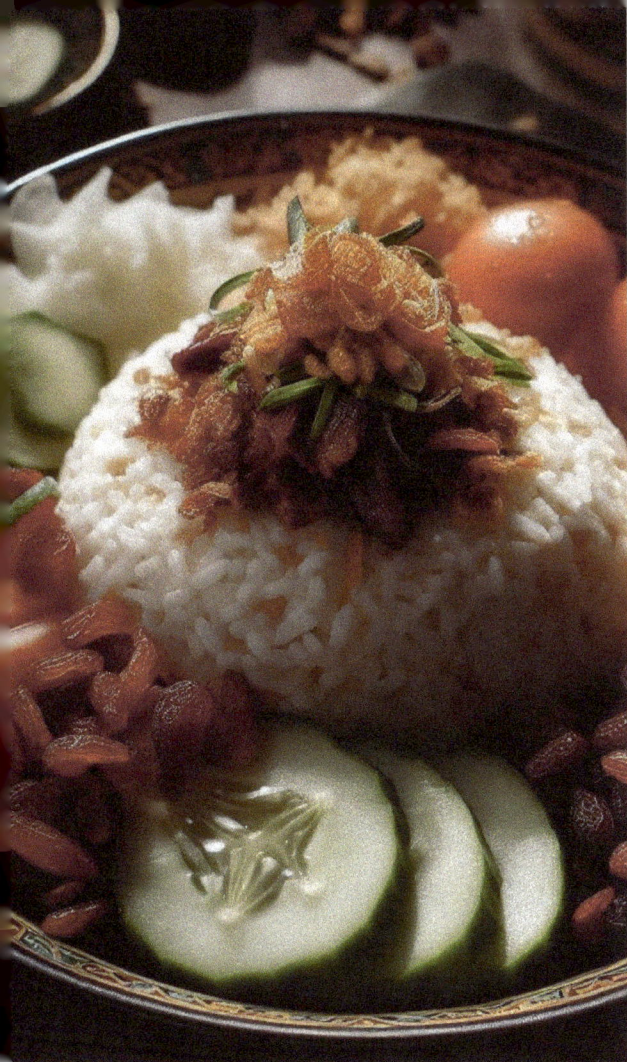

SPICED LAMB RICE (NASI KEBULI)

This dish is a mouthwatering and satisfying dish, full of nutrients!

TOTAL TIME 30-35 MINS **SERVINGS** 4

Instructions

1. In a large pot, heat the butter and sauté the sliced onion and minced garlic until fragrant.
2. Add the lamb or beef chunks and brown them on all sides.
3. Stir in the ground spices (cinnamon, cardamom, cloves), salt, and pepper.
4. Add the basmati rice and mix well.
5. Pour in the chicken or beef broth and bring to a boil.
6. Reduce the heat, cover, and simmer for about 20 minutes or until the rice is cooked and the meat is tender.

Ingredients

- 2 cups basmati rice
- 500g lamb (cut into chunks)
- 1 large onion (sliced)
- 4 cloves garlic (minced)
- 1 tsp ground cinnamon
- 1 tsp ground cardamom
- 1 tsp ground cloves
- Salt and pepper to taste
- 2 tbsp butter
- 4 cups chicken or beef broth

Notes:
- Mustaḥab foods included: rice, lamb, onion and garlic.

54

MORROCAN CHICKPEA TAGINE

This traditional meal is highly nutritious, filling while being light on the stomach.

PREP TIME
5 MINS

COOK TIME
30-40 MINS

SERVINGS
4

Instructions

1. In a large pot, sauté the chopped onion and minced garlic until fragrant.
2. Add the sliced carrots, zucchini, and red bell pepper.
3. Stir in the chickpeas, diced tomatoes, and spices (cumin, coriander, cinnamon, salt, and pepper).
4. Cover and simmer for about 30 minutes or until the vegetables are tender.
5. Garnish with fresh cilantro or parsley before serving. Serve with rice, quinoa or couscous.

Notes:
- Mustaḥab foods included: rice, chickpea, onion and garlic.

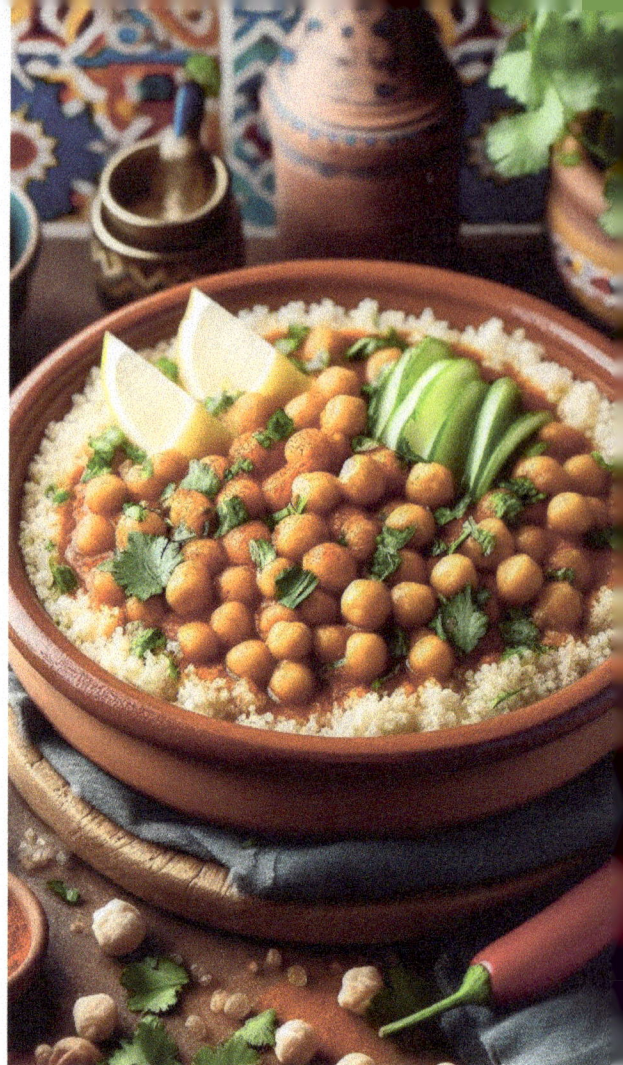

Ingredients

- 2 (15oz) cans chickpeas, drained and rinsed
- 1 large onion, chopped
- 3 garlic cloves, minced
- 2 large carrots, sliced
- 1 large zucchini, sliced
- 1 red bell pepper, sliced
- 1 can (14 oz) diced tomatoes
- 1 tsp ground cumin
- 1 tsp ground coriander
- ½ tsp ground cinnamon
- Salt and pepper to taste
- Fresh cilantro or parsley (chopped, for garnish)

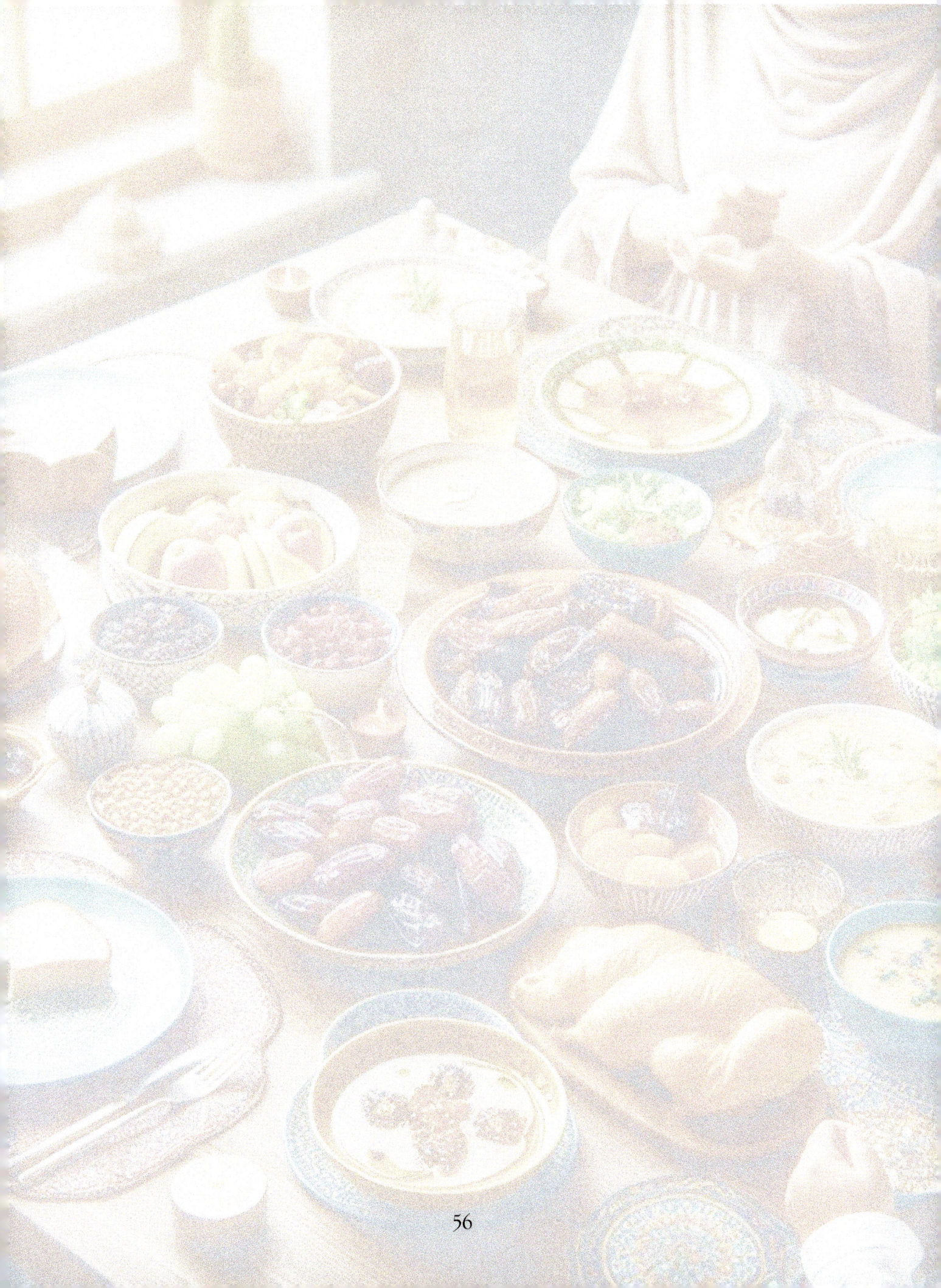

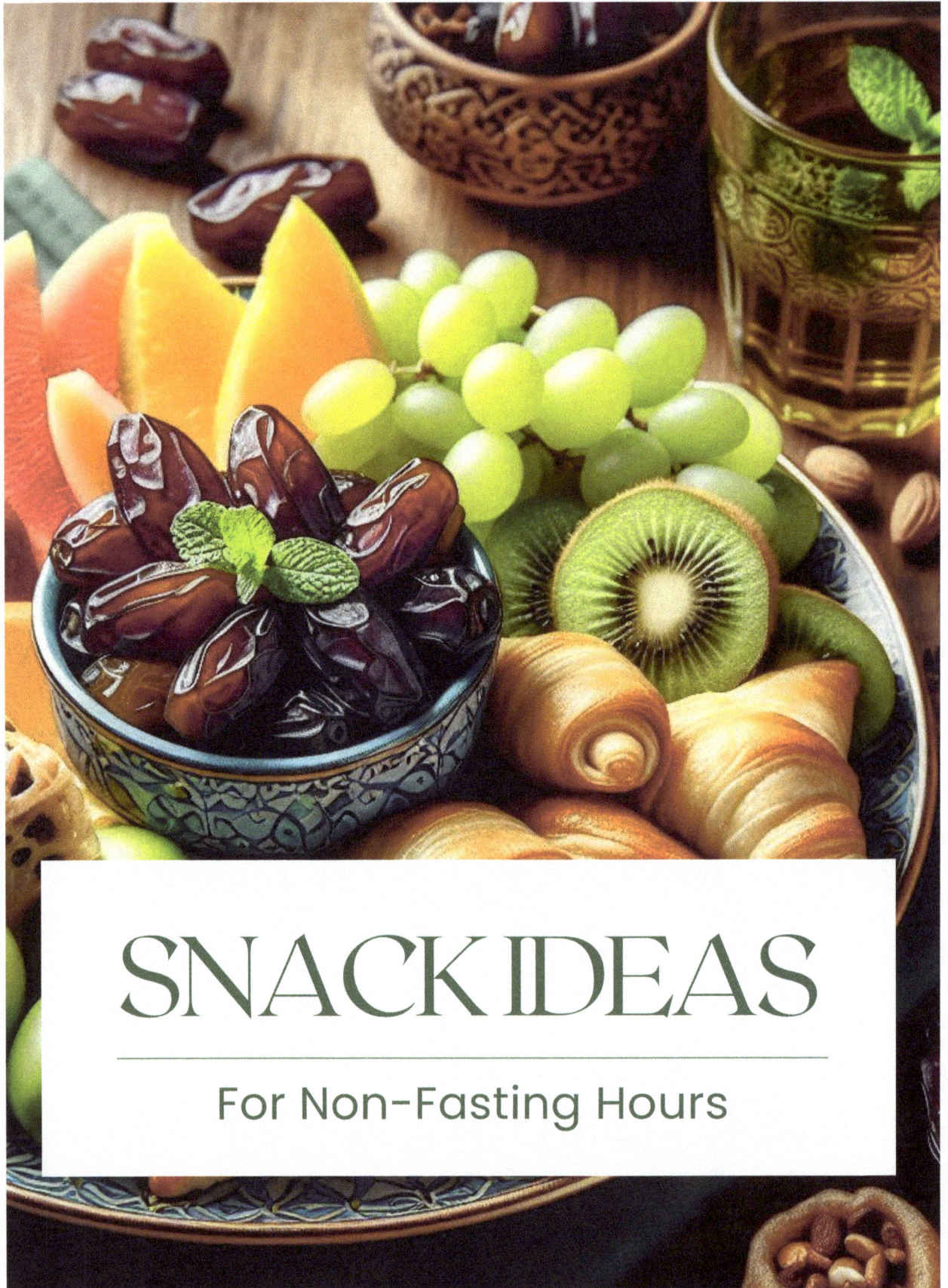

SNACK IDEAS

For Non-Fasting Hours

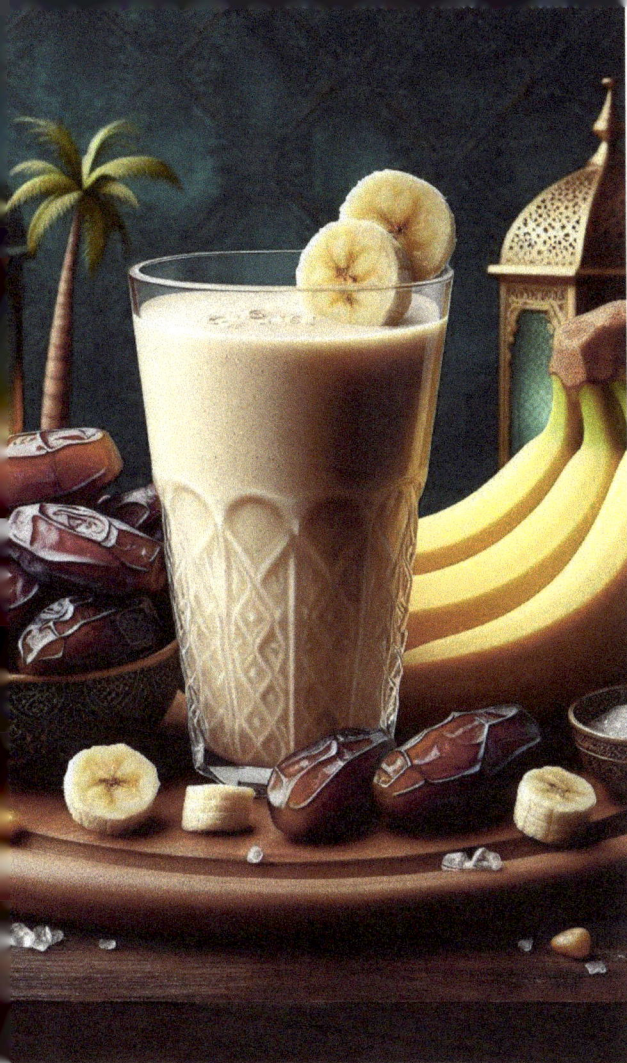

DATE AND BANANA SMOOTHIE

This sweet and creamy smoothie is rich in dietary fibre, a source of calcium, anti-oxidants as well as vitamins and minerals!

TOTAL TIME
5 MINS

SERVINGS
1 GLASS

Instructions

1. Add the milk, bananas, dates, honey, cinnamon, Greek yogurt, and ice cubes to a blender.
2. Blend on high speed until the mixture is smooth and creamy.
3. Pour into a glass and enjoy immediately.

Ingredients

- 1 cup milk (or a milk alternative like almond milk)
- 2 ripe bananas
- 4-5 dates, pitted
- 1 tbsp honey
- 1/2 tsp cinnamon
- 1/2 cup Greek yogurt
- A handful of ice cubes

Notes:
- Mustaḥab foods included: banana, dates, honey and yogurt.

ENERGY DATE BALLS

This is a wonderful snack providing you a natural boost of energy!

PREP TIME
5 MINS

COOK TIME
30-40 MINS

SERVINGS
4-6

Instructions

1. In a food processor, blend the pitted dates and almonds until they form a sticky mixture.
2. Add the shredded coconut, chia seeds, cocoa powder (if using), honey, vanilla extract, and a pinch of salt. Blend until well combined.
3. Scoop out small portions of the mixture and roll them into balls using your hands. If the mixture is too sticky, you can wet your hands slightly to make rolling easier.
4. Place the date balls on a plate or baking sheet and refrigerate for at least 30 minutes to firm up.
5. Store the energy date balls in an airtight container in the refrigerator. They can last for up to a week.

Notes:
- Mustaḥab foods included: dates, almonds and honey.

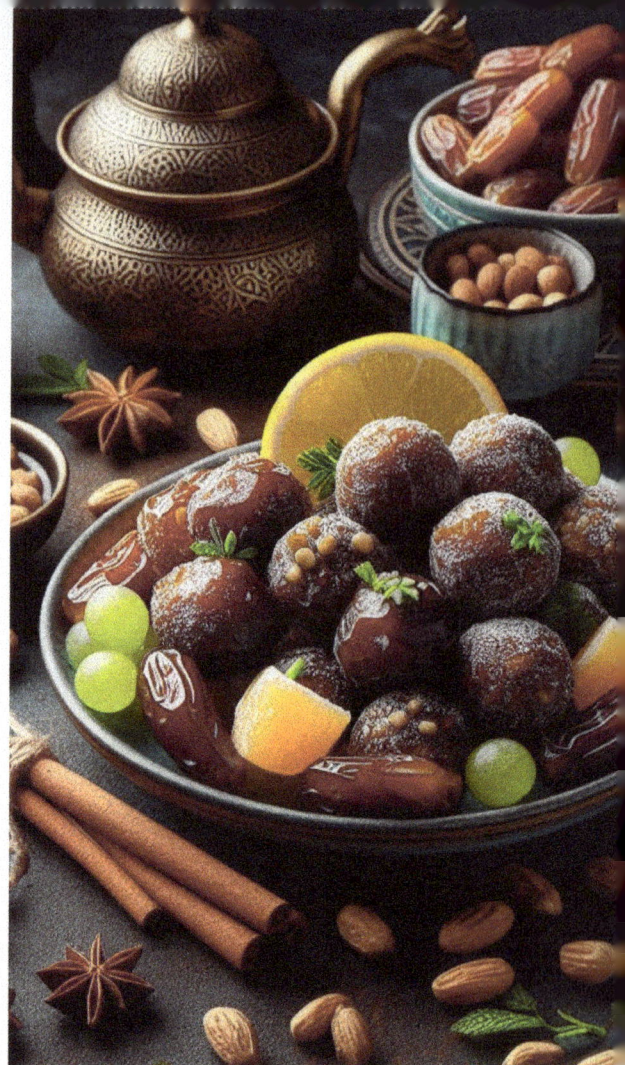

Ingredients

- 1 cup pitted dates
- 1/2 cup almonds (or any nuts of your choice)
- 1/4 cup shredded coconut
- 2 tbsp chia seeds
- 2 tbsp cocoa powder (optional, for a chocolatey flavour)
- 1 tbsp honey (optional, for extra sweetness)
- 1 tsp vanilla extract
- A pinch of salt

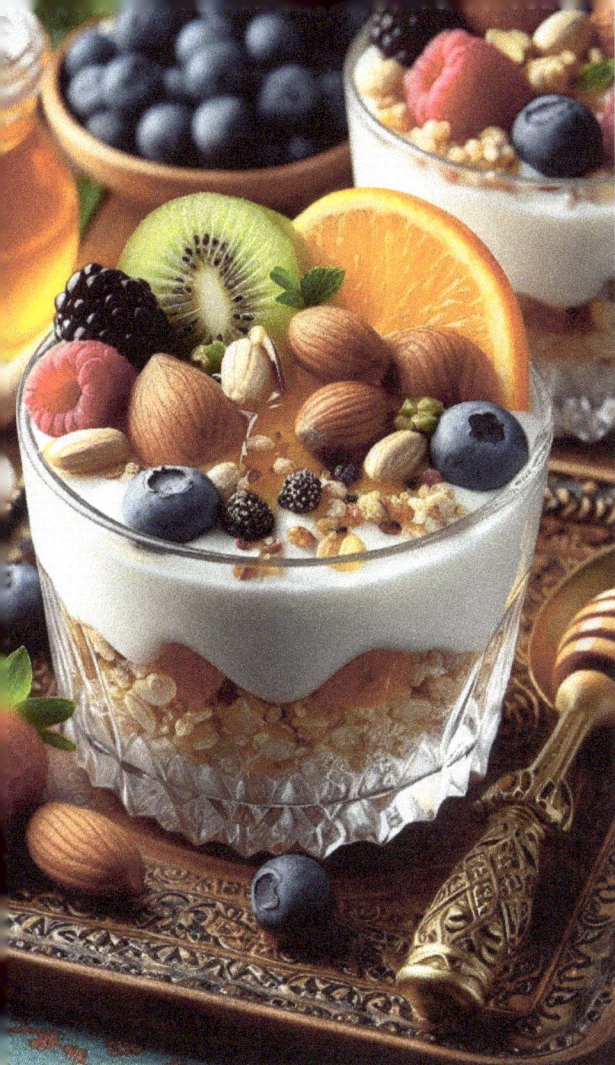

HONEY AND GREEK YOGURT PARFAIT

This wholesome snack is a great source of protein, probiotics with natural sweetness!

TOTAL TIME 7 MINS

SERVINGS 1 BOWL

Instructions

1. Place the Greek yogurt in a bowl or a glass.
2. Drizzle the honey over the yogurt.
3. Add the mixed fresh fruits on top of the yogurt.
4. Sprinkle the mixed nuts and seeds over the fruits.
5. Enjoy immediately as a delicious and nutritious snack.

Ingredients

- 1 cup Greek yogurt
- 1 tbsp honey
- 1/2 cup mixed fresh fruits
- 2 tbsp mixed nuts (like almonds, walnuts, or pistachios)
- 1 tbsp seeds (like chia seeds, flaxseeds, or sunflower seeds)

Notes:
- Mustaḥab foods included: yogurt, honey and fruits.
- Options for fruits to use can include berries, banana slices, apple cubes or any other fruits of your choice

VEGETABLE STICKS AND HUMMUS

⏱ TOTAL TIME **40 MINS** 🍽 SERVINGS **4**

Instructions

1. In a food processor, combine the tahini and lemon juice. Process for 1 minute, scrape the sides and bottom of the bowl, then process for 30 seconds more.
2. Add the olive oil, minced garlic, cumin, and a pinch of salt to the whipped tahini and lemon juice. Process for 30 seconds, scrape the sides and bottom of the bowl, then process for 30 seconds more.
3. Add half of the chickpeas to the food processor and process for 1 minute. Scrape the sides and bottom of the bowl, then add the remaining chickpeas and process until thick and smooth, 1 to 2 minutes.
4. With the food processor running, add 2 to 3 tablespoons of water until the hummus reaches your desired consistency.
5. Transfer the hummus to a serving bowl, drizzle with olive oil, and sprinkle with paprika.

Notes:
- Mustaḥab foods included: insert
- Vegetable options you can include could be carrots, celery, bell pepper etc.

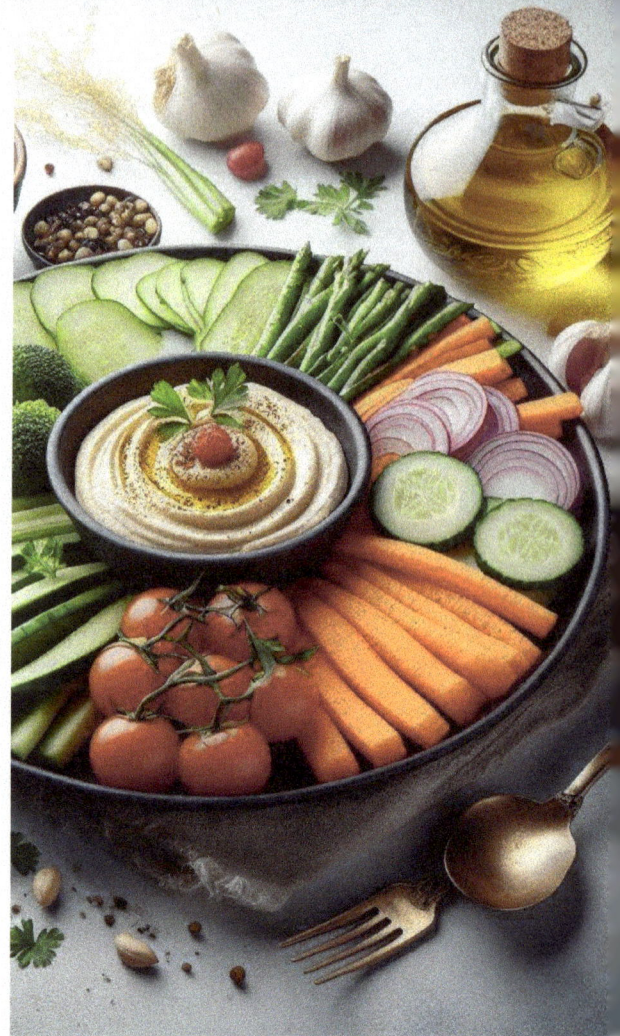

Ingredients

- **For Hummus:**
  - 1 can (15 oz) chickpeas, drained and rinsed
  - 1/4 cup lemon juice
  - 1/4 cup tahini
  - 1 small garlic clove, minced
  - 2 tbsp olive oil
  - 1/2 tsp ground cumin
  - Salt to taste
  - 2 to 3 tbsp water
  - Dash of ground paprika
- **Vegetables**
  - Any vegetables you like

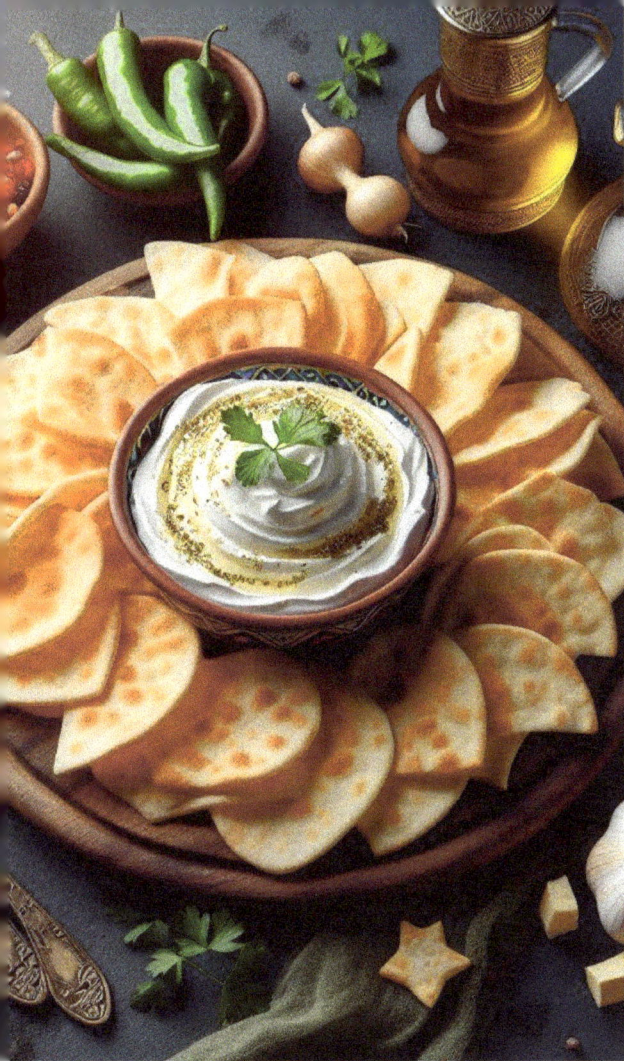

LABNEH WITH PITA

⏱ PREP TIME **30 MINS** ⏱ TOTAL TIME **30 MINS** 🍽 SERVINGS **4**

Instructions

1. Place your Greek yogurt/labneh into a plate.
2. Drizzle olive oil over the top.
3. Sprinkle with your spices if desired.
4. Cut the pita bread into wedges. Optionally, you can warm/crisp up the pita wedges in the oven for a few minutes.
5. Serve the labneh with the pita wedges on the side for dipping.

Ingredients

- 1 1/2 cup Greek yogurt or store-bought Labneh
- 1/2 teaspoon salt
- 1 tbsp olive oil
- 1 tsp of spices
  - Dried mint (optional)
  - Zaatar
  - Oregano
  - Paprika
  - Any spice you like
- Pita bread, cut into wedges

Notes:

- Mustaḥab foods included: yogurt, olive oil and bread.
- Add a drizzle of pomagrante mollasses on the labneh for some sweetness and tartness!

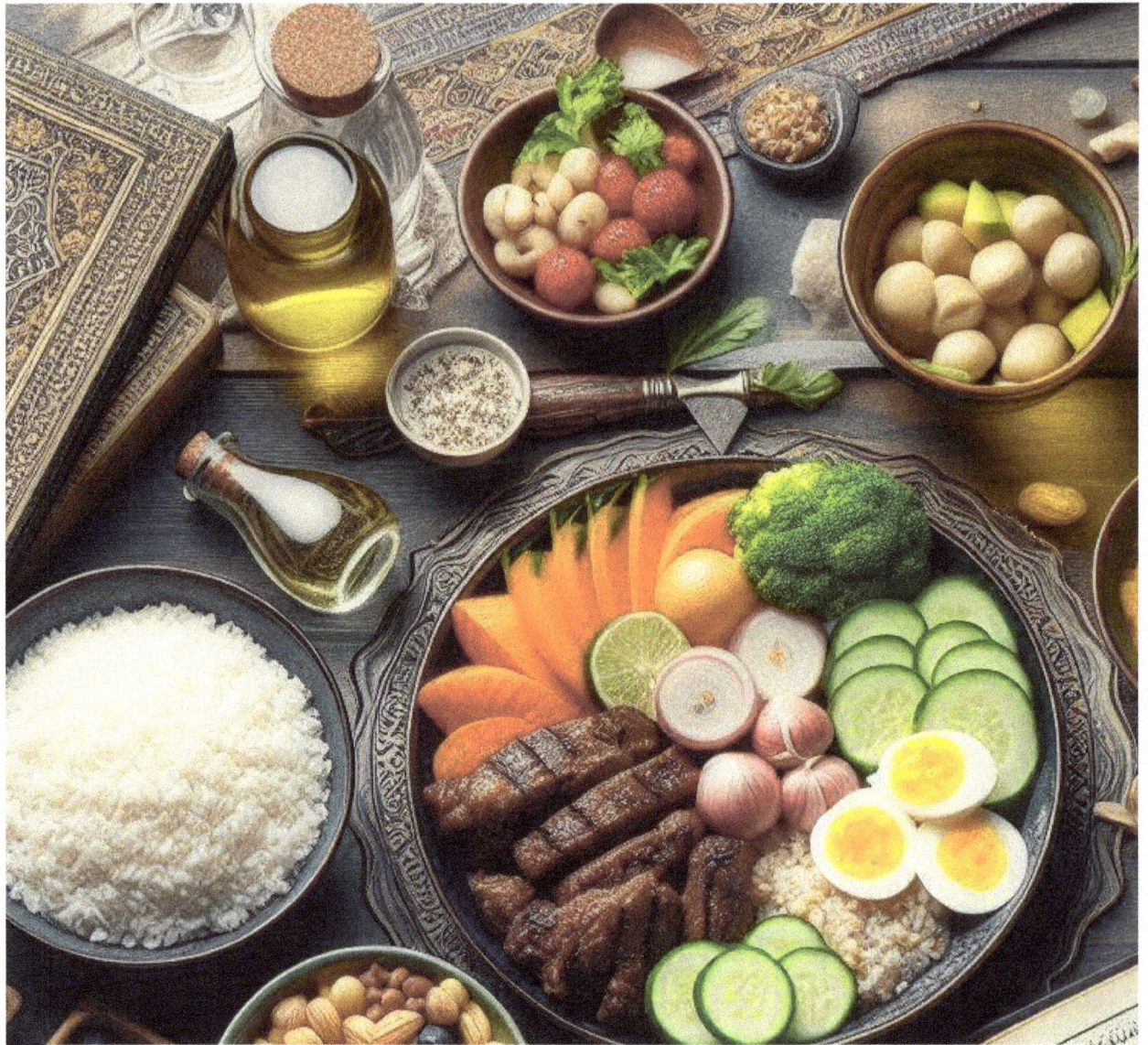

MEAL PLANNING

Tips for your busy lifestyle

MEAL PLANNING GUIDELINES

Balancing macronutrients—proteins, fats, and carbohydrates—is essential for maintaining energy levels and overall health during Shahr Ramaḍān.

PROTEINS	CARBOHYDRATES	FRUITS AND VEGETABLES	HEALTHY FATS
Chicken	Rice (preferably brown)	Apples	Olive Oil
Lamb	Quinoa	Berries	Avocados
Fish (tuna, salmon, white fish etc.)	Bread (whole wheat)	Dates	Nuts (Almonds, walnuts etc.)
Eggs, Yogurt	Oats	Carrots, Broccoli, Cucumber	Seeds (chia, flax, sesame and pumpkin)
Lentils, chickpeas	Couscous	Spinach	Nut butters (peanut, almond etc.)
Cheese	Pasta	Bell Peppers	Fatty fish (salmon etc.)

7 day MEAL PLAN

	SUḤŪR	IFṬĀR	SNACK
MON	An omelette made with eggs, spinach, tomatoes, bell peppers, and onions, served with whole-grain toast.	Grilled lamb with couscous, roasted bell peppers and a side of lentil soup	Vegetable sticks (cucumber, celery, carrots etc.) with Hummus
TUE	Greek yogurt parfait with honey, berries, and chia seeds	Grilled chicken with quinoa, steamed broccoli, and a tzatziki dip	Dates with a side of nuts (almonds, cashews, pecans etc.)
WED	Scrambled eggs with spinach and whole wheat toast	Baked salmon with sweet potatoes and a spinach salad with avocado slices	Smoothie with Greek yogurt, dates and frozen fruits.
THU	Labneh drizzled with olive oil and served with whole wheat pita bread and a side of olives and cucumbers.	Baked fish with barley and a side of steamed vegetables	Date Energy Balls

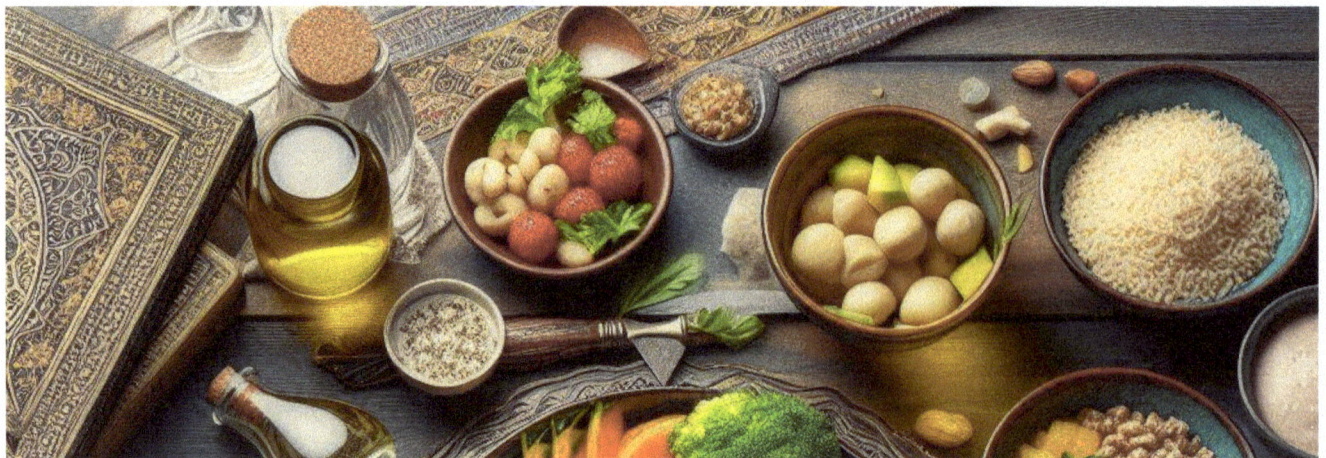

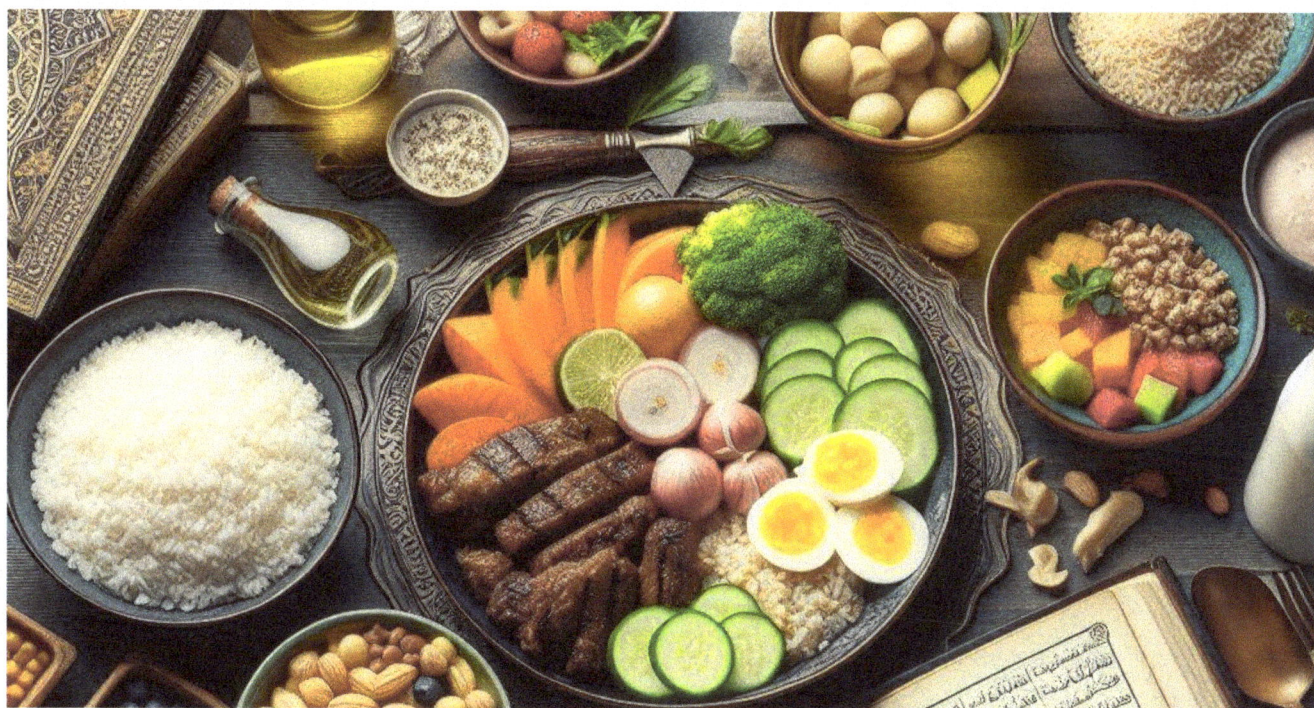

	SUḤŪR	IFṬĀR	SNACK
FRI	Whole grain toast topped with mashed avocado and a poached or scrambled egg.	Bell peppers stuffed with a mixture of minced meat (lamb, beef or chicken), black beans, corn, tomatoes, and spices. Side of pasta salad	Homemade trail mix with dried fruits (cranberries, blueberries, strawberries etc.), dates, nuts (almonds, peanuts etc.) and seeds (sunflower, pumpkin etc.)
SAT	Greek yogurt parfait with oats, chia seeds, and a drizzle of honey	Grilled chicken wrapped in whole wheat pita with lettuce, tomatoes, cucumbers, and a drizzle of tahini sauce. Side of Hummus.	Smoothie with Greek yogurt, berries, spinach, and a tablespoon of flaxseeds.
SUN	Oatmeal cooked with broth, topped with sautéed spinach, mushrooms, and a poached egg.	Grilled chicken and vegetable (bell peppers, onions, tomato and zucchini) skewers, served with a side of couscous or quinoa.	Cream cheese and spice stuffed baby bell peppers

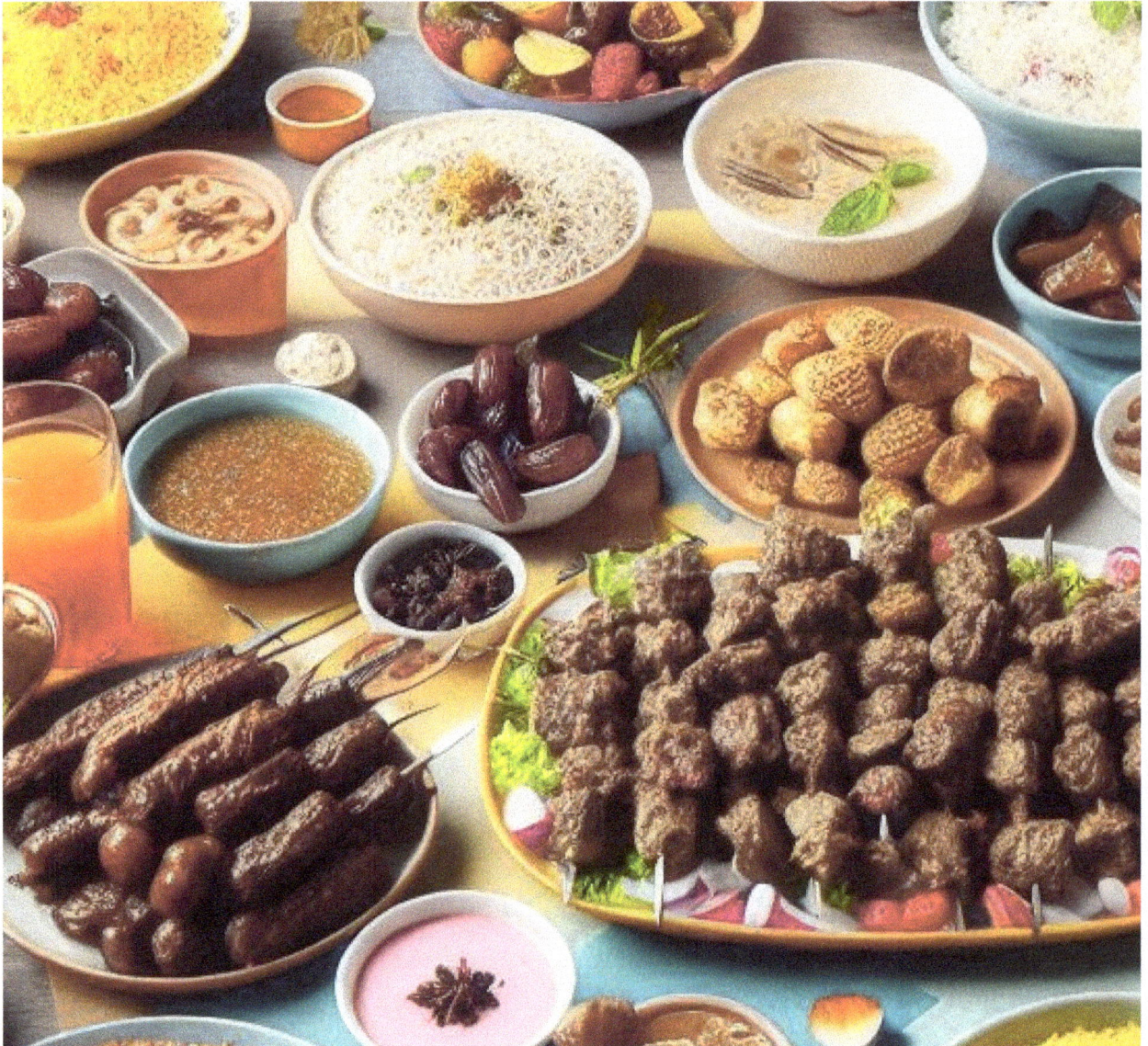

POST SHAHR
RAMAḌAN

Adjusting after a month of fasting

Transitioning BACK INTO NON-FASTING EATING HABITS

1 **Light Meals**:
Start with <u>lighter meals</u> and maintain this approach to avoid overwhelming your digestive system.

2 **Balanced Meals**:
Focus on meals that include protein, carbohydrates, and healthy fats, along with plenty of fruits and vegetables. This will help in <u>maintaining energy levels</u> and <u>supporting overall health</u>.

3 **Mindful Eating**:
Pay attention to hunger and fullness cues! <u>Eat slowly and savour your food</u> to improve digestion.

4 **Healthy Snacking**:
Incorporate snacks like nuts, seeds, fruits, and yogurt to <u>keep your energy levels stable</u> between meals.

HABITS TO KEEP

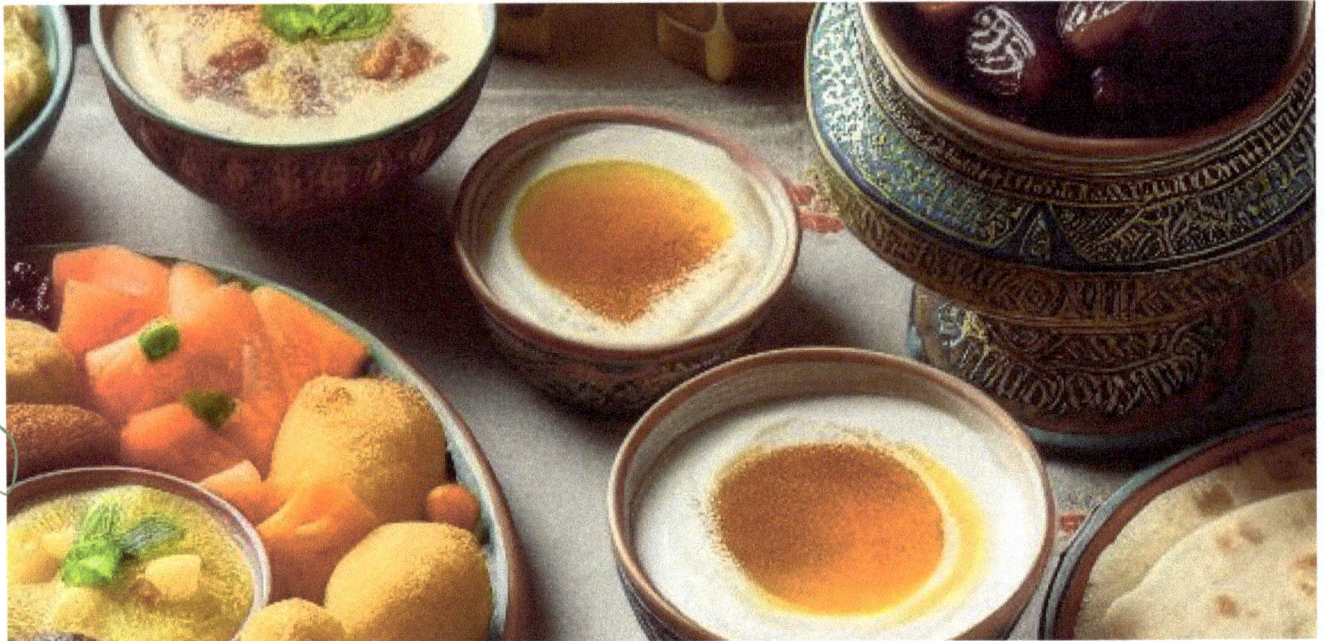

- **Occasional fasting**: <u>Fast</u> every once in a while, especially on the recommended days (Mondays, Thursdays, the 13th, 14th and 15th days of every lunar month etc.).
- **Regular Meal Times**: Try to <u>stick to regular meal times</u> to help regulate your body's internal clock and improve digestion.
- **Nutrient-Dense Foods**: Continue to <u>choose nutrient-dense foods</u> like whole grains, lean proteins, healthy fats, and a variety of fruits and vegetables.
- **Hydration**: Keep up with <u>good hydration</u> habits by drinking water regularly throughout the day.
- **Physical Activity:** Incorporate <u>regular physical activity</u> into your routine to support overall health and well-being.